Andrews' Diseases of the Skin
Clinical Atlas

Andrews' Diseases of the Skin
CLINICAL ATLAS

William D. James, MD
Paul R. Gross Professor of Dermatology
Department of Dermatology
Perelman School of Medicine at the University of Pennsylvania
Philadelphia
Pennsylvania
USA

Dirk M. Elston, MD
Professor and Chairman
Department of Dermatology and Dermatologic Surgery
Medical University of South Carolina
Charleston
South Carolina
USA

Patrick J. McMahon, MD
Assistant Professor of Pediatrics and Dermatology at The Children's Hospital of Philadelphia and University of Pennsylvania School of Medicine
Philadelphia
Pennsylvania
USA

ELSEVIER

For additional online content visit
ExpertConsult.com

Edinburgh   London   New York   Oxford   Philadelphia   St Louis   Sydney   Toronto   2018

ELSEVIER

© 2018, Elsevier Inc. All rights reserved.

No part of this publication may be reproduced or transmitted in any form or by any means, electronic or mechanical, including photocopying, recording, or any information storage and retrieval system, without permission in writing from the publisher. Details on how to seek permission, further information about the Publisher's permissions policies and our arrangements with organizations such as the Copyright Clearance Center and the Copyright Licensing Agency, can be found at our website: www.elsevier.com/permissions.

This book and the individual contributions contained in it are protected under copyright by the Publisher (other than as may be noted herein).

Notices

Knowledge and best practice in this field are constantly changing. As new research and experience broaden our understanding, changes in research methods, professional practices, or medical treatment may become necessary.

Practitioners and researchers must always rely on their own experience and knowledge in evaluating and using any information, methods, compounds, or experiments described herein. In using such information or methods they should be mindful of their own safety and the safety of others, including parties for whom they have a professional responsibility.

With respect to any drug or pharmaceutical products identified, readers are advised to check the most current information provided (i) on procedures featured or (ii) by the manufacturer of each product to be administered, to verify the recommended dose or formula, the method and duration of administration, and contraindications. It is the responsibility of practitioners, relying on their own experience and knowledge of their patients, to make diagnoses, to determine dosages and the best treatment for each individual patient, and to take all appropriate safety precautions.

To the fullest extent of the law, neither the Publisher nor the authors, contributors, or editors, assume any liability for any injury and/or damage to persons or property as a matter of products liability, negligence or otherwise, or from any use or operation of any methods, products, instructions, or ideas contained in the material herein.

ISBN: 978-0-323-44196-4

Executive Content Strategist: Russell Gabbedy
Content Development Specialist: Carole McMurray
Project Manager: Julie Taylor
Design: Christian Bilbow
Illustration Manager: Karen Giacomucci
Illustrator: Graphic World
Marketing Manager: Kristin Koehler

your source for books, journals and multimedia in the health sciences
www.elsevierhealth.com

Working together to grow libraries in developing countries
www.elsevier.com • www.bookaid.org

The publisher's policy is to use paper manufactured from sustainable forests

Printed in China
Last digit is the print number: 9 8 7 6 5 4 3 2

CONTENTS

Preface		vi
Dedication		vii

1. Structure and Function — 1
2. Cutaneous Signs and Diagnosis — 15
3. Dermatoses Resulting from Physical Factors — 27
4. Pruritus and Neurocutaneous Diseases — 41
5. Atopic Dermatitis, Eczema, and Noninfectious Immunodeficiency Disorders — 53
6. Contact Dermatitis and Drug Eruptions — 65
7. Erythema and Urticaria — 87
8. Connective Tissue Diseases — 101
9. Mucinoses — 119
10. Seborrheic Dermatitis, Psoriasis, Recalcitrant Palmoplantar Eruptions, Pustular Dermatitis, and Erythroderma — 125
11. Pityriasis Rosea, Pityriasis Rubra Pilaris, and Other Papulosquamous and Hyperkeratotic Diseases — 139
12. Lichen Planus and Related Conditions — 153
13. Acne — 169
14. Bacterial Infections — 185
15. Diseases Resulting from Fungi and Yeasts — 203
16. Mycobacterial Diseases — 229
17. Hansen Disease — 239
18. Syphilis, Yaws, Bejel, and Pinta — 251
19. Viral Diseases — 263
20. Parasitic Infestations, Stings, and Bites — 291
21. Chronic Blistering Dermatoses — 309
22. Nutritional Diseases — 323
23. Diseases of Subcutaneous Fat — 331
24. Endocrine Diseases — 339
25. Abnormalities of Dermal Fibrous and Elastic Tissue — 351
26. Errors in Metabolism — 361
27. Genodermatoses and Congenital Anomalies — 379
28. Dermal and Subcutaneous Tumors — 405
29. Epidermal Nevi, Neoplasms, and Cysts — 437
30. Melanocytic Nevi and Neoplasms — 463
31. Macrophage/Monocyte Disorders — 479
32. Cutaneous Lymphoid Hyperplasia, Cutaneous T-Cell Lymphoma, Other Malignant Lymphomas, and Allied Diseases — 501
33. Diseases of Skin Appendages — 517
34. Diseases of Mucous Membranes — 543
35. Cutaneous Vascular Diseases — 561
36. Disturbances of Pigmentation — 583

Index — 595

PREFACE

It is our pleasure to bring to you this atlas of skin disorders. We are hopeful that by seeing this wide array of images you may better recognize and diagnose skin conditions in your own patients. If our efforts result in a better outcome of one patient, then this was worthwhile. Our atlas is an accompanying volume to *Andrews' Diseases of the Skin*. The chapters and entities follow the organization of our Andrews' text, making explanatory text unnecessary, allowing you to simply enjoy the superior photographs in an uncluttered fashion.

Dermatologic diagnostic abilities are learned through repetitive exposures to patient presentations. The present volume of over 3000 pictures, combined with the main textbook, will be an outstanding resource to learn the depth and breadth of our specialty.

The three authors have benefitted by spending a combined 50 years in academic medicine, taking photographs along the journey. Additionally the resources of our institutions and many friends made this a book that allows a stunning array and variety of presentations to be represented. Bill James recognizes Richard Odom, MD, my teaching chief, who allowed myself and fellow resident Robert Horn to make copies of his best slides. Tim Berger has shared photographs from his experiences at the University of California at San Francisco. The faculty and residents at both Walter Reed Army Medical Center and the University of Pennsylvania have also generously shared their expertise. Dirk thanks those members of Brooke Army Medical Center who have contributed to the image collection in San Antonio, as well as the faculty and residents at the Rutgers Robert Wood Johnson School of Medicine. Finally, Pat wishes to gratefully recognize that the considerable resources of Drs. Paul Honig and Walter Tunnessen's personal collections were made fully available. Additionally, the combined image database of the current pediatric dermatology faculty at The Children's Hospital of Philadelphia (Albert Yan, MD; James Treat, MD; Leslie, Castelo, MD; Melinda Jen, MD; and Marissa Perman, MD) was utilized to enhance this atlas considerably. Finally, James Fitzpatrick, MD, also generously shared photographs taken by the faculty and staff of Fitzsimmons Army Medical Center. We call out all of these wonderful people as they are not recognized individually in most of the photographs. In some cases where a specific photograph was obtained from a specific faculty or resident, their names appear in a "Courtesy" line under the image.

You will find over 50 individuals recognized in the figure legends. These range from institutions in Brazil and Japan, to individuals in Singapore, India, and the Philippines, to the National Institutes of Health, the University of Pennsylvania School of Dental Medicine, and faculty from a variety of academic centers around the country. Several individuals deserve special mention: Steven Binnick, MD, is a superb dermatologist practicing in Plymouth Meeting, Pennsylvania. When Bill asked if he would make available some of his excellent photographs for this atlas, he simply donated his collection and was happy they would be used to educate others. Curt Samlaska, MD, trained at Walter Reed with Bill. He is an outstanding dermatologic photographer and contributed many photos of his patients from Hawaii and his practice in Henderson, Nevada. The late Don Adler, MD, was a friend who shared with Bill many photos over the years. Some of his superior images are part of this work. Shyam Verma, MD, a close friend from India, shared many of his wonderful images from his private practice. Debabrata Bandyopadhyay, MD, also provided special pictures of rare conditions from the Medical College in Kolkata. Scott Norton, MD, shared many photographs from his wide experience at Fitzsimmons, Walter Reed, and the Children's National Health System. Len Sperling, MD, has always generously contributed images of hair disorders, both for this volume and for prior Andrews' textbooks.

This wide array of altruistic physicians and many others individually recognized in the atlas under their photos allows us to demonstrate entities rarely or never seen in the United States. More importantly is the full spectrum of ages, skin types, subtypes of diseases, morphologies, and highly representative classic examples that were available for us to choose only the best 3000+ images that make up this volume.

Bill, Dirk, and Pat also want to highlight the steadfast, expert assistance of Barbara Lang in bringing this volume to fruition. She made the work move along in an organized manner, paying attention to all the details along the way. The images were expertly handled by Elsevier through Graphic World, as many photos were in slide form and needed scanning. Mark Lane, Patty Bassman, and Cindy Geiss deserve special recognition, and Karen Giacomucci with Elsevier in Philadelphia assumed overall responsibility for coordinating this aspect of the work. Carole McMurray and Julie Taylor from the British offices of Elsevier assumed primary roles in the compilation of the book. Russell Gabbedy has been our now-constant companion from Elsevier in not only enabling this atlas to be supported, but also working with us on prior editions of the main text *Andrews' Diseases of the Skin*.

No words of thanks could be complete without acknowledging the personal sacrifices of our families in allowing us the opportunity to pursue our professional dreams. Those include all of the individuals listed in the dedication.

Bill James, Dirk Elston and Patrick McMahon

DEDICATION

Bill James, Dirk Elston, Patrick McMahon

To my loving family:

My wife Ann, son Dan, daughter Becca, daughter-in-law Wynn, grandsons Declan and Driscoll, and sister Judy and her husband Cal.
You have given me a wonderful life!
Bill James

To my wife Kathy and my children, Carly and Nate. You make the world a wonderful place.
Dirk Elston

To my amazing wife, Kate, and wonderful children, Bridget, Brendan, Colin, and Molly.
Thank you for the love, the laughs, and the support.
You fill every day with joy!
Patrick McMahon

To all of our past patients, we hope this work fulfills your desire to help future sufferers of skin disease to recover more rapidly through early recognition of their condition.
Bill, Dirk, and Pat

Structure and Function

1

The diagnosis of skin disease is based on color, morphology, and distribution of cutaneous lesions. The structure of the skin and associated appendages relates directly to these characteristics.

Folliculitis presents with papules or pustules. Follicular accentuation is characteristic of any eruption in darker-skinned races. In patients with miliaria, involvement of the sweat gland ostia results in erythematous papules, pustules, or superficial vesicles in areas of heavy sweating. The vesicles of miliaria crystallina are irregular in shape because the stratum corneum fails to impede the spread of the blister in random directions. This is in stark contrast to spongiotic and subepidermal blisters, which are distinctly round—as in acute dyshidrotic eczema or bullous pemphigoid.

The color of a cutaneous eruption relates to various pigments. Brown pigments include melanin, lipofuscin, and hemosiderin. Brown pigments located deeper in the dermis impart a blue hue because of diffraction of light. This is evident in blue nevi as a result of deep melanin and as a result of lipofuscin present in the sweat within nodular hidradenomas. Red pigment relates to oxygenated hemoglobin and blue to deoxygenated hemoglobin. Dilatation or proliferation of blood vessels and the rapidity of blood flow produce various shades of red and blue. Yellow pigments relate to lipid deposition or carotenoids dissolved in the cytoplasm of epithelial cells and histiocytes. In granulomatous disease, diascopy removes the visible appearance of oxygenated hemoglobin, allowing the observer to see the apple jelly yellow appearance of carotenoids within the cytoplasm. This section of the atlas will focus on the structure of the skin and how that structure translates to clinical manifestations of disease.

Fig. 1.1 In early fetal life, a cuboidal periderm is present, rather than an epidermis. Fetal skin, H&E × 40.

Fig. 1.2 In early fetal life, the spine is composed of cartilage, and mesenchyme is present rather than a dermis. Mesenchyme heals without scar formation. Once dermis forms, scars will occur after injury. Fetal skin, H&E × 40.

Fig. 1.3 Skin in young children is characterized by small adnexal structures and fine dermal collagen bundles that stain deep red in contrast to the thick, pink collagen bundles of an adult. Many plump fibroblasts are present in the dermis, actively synthesizing collagen. Childhood skin, H&E × 20.

Fig. 1.4 Facial skin is characterized by prominent sebaceous follicles, often containing *Demodex* mites. Facial skin, H&E × 40.

Fig. 1.5 Skin of the ear demonstrates small adnexal structures with an elastic cartilage surrounded by a red perichondrium. Ear skin, H&E × 20.

Fig. 1.6 The structure of the ear canal is similar to other parts of the ear, except for the presence of ceruminous glands, which represent modified apocrine glands. Ear canal skin, H&E × 20.

Fig. 1.7 Scalp skin demonstrates many terminal hair follicles. The inferior segment of each follicle sits within the subcutaneous fat. Scalp skin, H&E × 40.

Fig. 1.8 Axillary skin is rugose and demonstrates large apocrine glands. Axillary skin, H&E × 40.

Fig. 1.9 Breast skin demonstrates numerous smooth muscle bundles. Breast skin, H&E × 20.

Fig. 1.10 Nipple skin demonstrates smaller smooth muscle bundles. The mammary duct resembles a large sweat duct. Breast skin, H&E × 20.

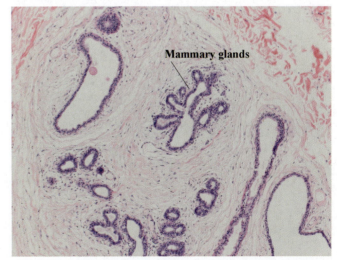

Fig. 1.11 The secretory portion of mammary glands demonstrates columnar epithelium forming complex lumens. Breast skin, H&E × 100.

Fig. 1.12 Prepuce demonstrates a rugose appearance with many smooth muscle fascicles and high vascularity. Prepuce, H&E × 20.

Fig. 1.14 The lid margin; on the cutaneous surface of the lid, a layer of striated muscle is present below the epidermis, H&E × 10.

Fig. 1.13 Eyelid anatomy, below the conjunctiva; the densely fibrous tarsal plate contains sebaceous glands (meibomian glands), H&E × 100.

Fig. 1.15 Volar skin demonstrates a thick stratum corneum and lack of hair follicles, low power, H&E × 40.

Fig. 1.16 Volar skin demonstrating a thick corneum and dermis, H&E × 100.

Fig. 1.17 Volar skin, with deep tissue demonstrating Pacinian corpuscles, H&E × 100.

Fig. 1.18 Mucosal surface demonstrating nonkeratinizing epithelium and submucosa, H&E × 200.

Fig. 1.19 Below the epidermis, the papillary dermis is composed of fine, nonbundled collagen. Capillaries are present within the papillary dermis, and the postcapillary venule sits at the junction of the papillary and reticular dermis. H&E × 40.

Fig. 1.20 The lobules of the subcutaneous fat are separated by fibrous septae. H&E × 40.

Fig. 1.21 Hair anatomy, vertical, H&E × 200.

Fig. 1.22 In the inferior segment, the hair bulb gives rise to the inner and outer root sheath, H&E × 200.

Fig. 1.23 Hair anatomy, transverse, H&E × 200.

Fig. 1.24 Desmosome: A classic desmosome showing the following features: (i) Uniform gap of 20 to 30 nm between the apposed trilaminar plasma membranes with an intermediate line (*arrow*) in this gap. (ii) Sharply delineated dense plaques into which tonofibrils (F) converge. *Courtesy of Sunita Bhuta, MD.*

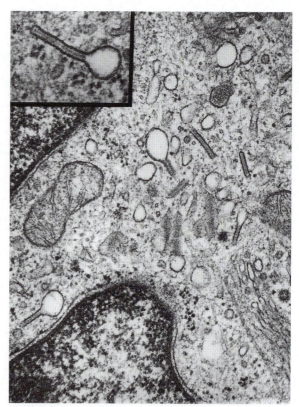

Fig. 1.25 Langerhans cell with Birbeck granules. This electromicrograph shows characteristic racket-shaped profiles of the granules in the cytoplasm (inset with higher magnification of the Birbeck granule). *Courtesy of Sunita Bhuta, MD.*

Fig. 1.26 Premelanosome: Solitary melanosome with characteristic internal striated structure. *Courtesy of Sunita Bhuta, MD.*

Fig. 1.27 Tonofibrils: Tonofibrils (intermediate filaments) lying free in the cytoplasm of a squamous cell. *Courtesy of Sunita Bhuta, MD.*

Fig. 1.28 Eosinophil: (A) Binucleate (N) with intracytoplasmic specific granules. (B) Specific granules have a finely granular matrix and a crystalline core. *Courtesy of Sunita Bhuta, MD.*

Fig. 1.29 Mast cell: Mast cell with numerous electron-dense granules. The inset shows internal structure of granules with membranous whorls (scrolls). *Courtesy of Sunita Bhuta, MD.*

Fig. 1.30 Merkel cell: Merkel cell with intracytoplasmic membrane bound, electron-dense granules with a halo (neurosecretory granules). *Courtesy of Sunita Bhuta, MD.*

Fig. 1.31 Skin tension lines relate to creases visible in older skin. They relate to passive skin tension, as well as active contraction of superficial muscular aponeurotic system muscle. Optimal surgical results can be achieved by aligning incisions along these lines.

Fig. 1.32 Skin tension lines on the trunk.

Fig. 1.33 Skin tension lines on the extremities.

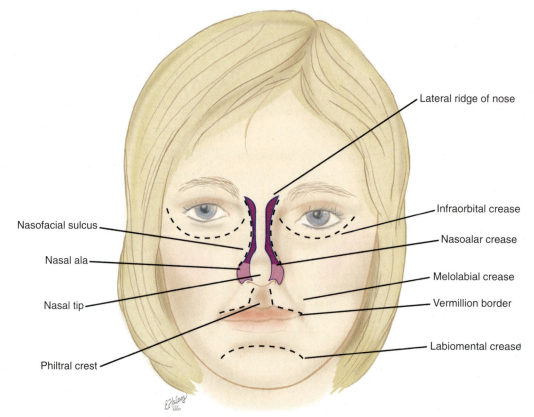

Fig. 1.34 Major anatomic landmarks.

Fig. 1.35 Anatomy of the ear, superficial temporal artery, and auriculotemporal nerve. *Courtesy Joseph F. Greco, MD and Christopher Skvarka, MD.*

Fig. 1.36 Anatomy of the parotid gland and related structures. *Courtesy Joseph F. Greco, MD and Christopher Skvarka, MD.*

Fig. 1.37 Anatomy of the parotid duct and facial nerve. *Courtesy Joseph F. Greco, MD and Christopher Skvarka, MD.*

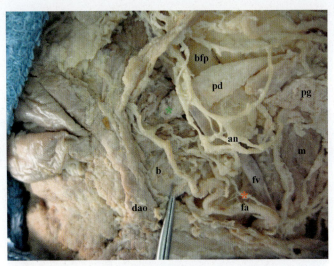

Fig. 1.38 Parotid duct as it pierces the buccinators muscle. *Courtesy Joseph F. Greco, MD and Christopher Skvarka, MD.*

Fig. 1.39 Superficial muscular aponeurotic system. *Courtesy Joseph F. Greco, MD and Christopher Skvarka, MD.*

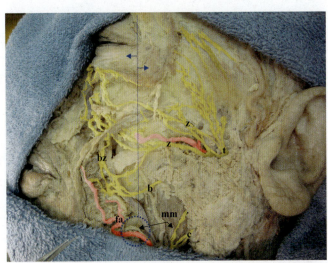

Fig. 1.40 Anatomy of the facial nerve. *Courtesy Joseph F. Greco, MD and Christopher Skvarka, MD.*

Fig. 1.41 The facial nerve: Danger zone for dermatologic surgery. *Courtesy Joseph F. Greco, MD and Christopher Skvarka, MD.*

Fig. 1.42 Muscles of facial expression. *Courtesy Joseph F. Greco, MD and Christopher Skvarka, MD.*

Structure and function

11

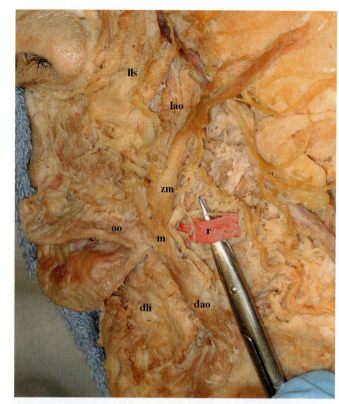

Fig. 1.43 Modiolus, elevators, and depressors. *Courtesy Joseph F. Greco, MD and Christopher Skvarka, MD.*

Fig. 1.45 Levator palpebrae superioris. *Courtesy Joseph F. Greco, MD and Christopher Skvarka, MD.*

Fig. 1.44 Innervation of the facial skin. *Courtesy Joseph F. Greco, MD and Christopher Skvarka, MD.*

Fig. 1.46 Medial forehead: Supraorbital and supratrochlear neurovascular structures. *Courtesy Joseph F. Greco, MD and Christopher Skvarka, MD.*

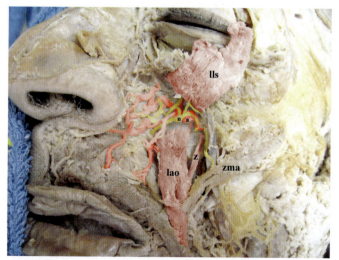

Fig. 1.47 Infraorbital foramen and related structures. *Courtesy Joseph F. Greco, MD and Christopher Skvarka, MD.*

Fig. 1.48 Mental foramen and related structures. *Courtesy Joseph F. Greco, MD and Christopher Skvarka, MD.*

Fig. 1.49 Anatomy of the posterior triangle of the neck (Erb point). *Courtesy Joseph F. Greco, MD and Christopher Skvarka, MD.*

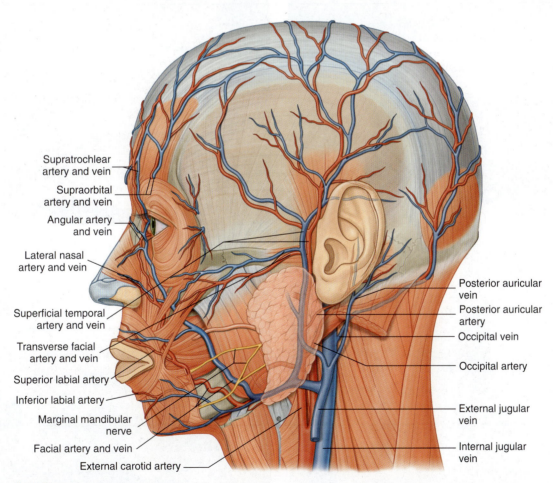

Fig. 1.50 Arterial and venous supply of the face.

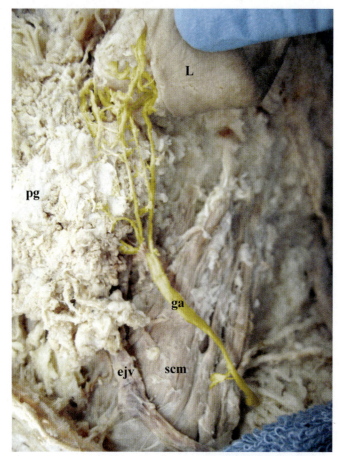

Fig. 1.51 Great auricular nerve and external jugular vein. *Courtesy Joseph F. Greco, MD and Christopher Skvarka, MD.*

Fig. 1.52 Facial artery with angular artery. *Courtesy Joseph F. Greco, MD and Christopher Skvarka, MD.*

Fig. 1.53 Inferior labial artery and related structures of the lower lip and chin. *Courtesy Joseph F. Greco, MD and Christopher Skvarka, MD.*

Fig. 1.54 Superior labial artery and related structures of the upper lip and cheek. *Courtesy Joseph F. Greco, MD and Christopher Skvarka, MD.*

Fig. 1.55 Layers of the scalp. *Courtesy Joseph F. Greco, MD and Christopher Skvarka, MD.*

Cutaneous Signs and Diagnosis

The astute clinician uses the appearance of the eruption and its accompanying symptoms to arrive at an accurate diagnosis. A symptom, such as itch or pain, is something that the patient reports. In contrast, a sign is elicited by the physician during examination. Pain is a symptom; tenderness to palpation is a sign.

This chapter will focus on the morphologic patterns skin lesions may have primarily or acquire over the course of time. The latter are called *secondary characteristics* and are not as helpful diagnostically as those present at the onset of the condition. Examples of each primary and secondary lesion are included, as well as other findings that are utilized to narrow the differential diagnosis such as the configuration, grouping, and color.

Finally, examples throughout will emphasize that the astute clinician should utilize all observable findings, inducing those of the hair, nails, and mucous membranes.

Fig. 2.1 Nevus of ota (macule). *Courtesy Steven Binnick, MD.*

Fig. 2.3 Voriconazole-induced lentigines (macules). *Courtesy Jennifer Huang, MD.*

Fig. 2.2 Axillary freckling neurofibromatosis (macules).

Fig. 2.4 Vitiligo (patch).

Fig. 2.5 Nevus depigmentosus (patch). *Courtesy Scott Norton, MD.*

Fig. 2.6 Drug eruption (macules, some small papules present surmounting the erythema).

Fig. 2.7 Drug eruption (morbilliform appearance).

Fig. 2.8 Sarcoidosis (papules).

Fig. 2.9 Eruptive xanthomas (papules). Yellow color is uncommon in the skin and helps to narrow the differential diagnosis.

Fig. 2.10 Darier disease (papules).

Fig. 2.11 Verruca vulgaris (scaly papule).

Fig. 2.12 Hypertrophic lupus erythematosus (scaly papules and plaques). *Courtesy Steven Binnick, MD.*

Fig. 2.13 Oral hairy leukoplakia (plaques).

Fig. 2.14 Psoriasis (plaques). *Courtesy Steven Binnick, MD.*

Fig. 2.15 Xanthomas in homozygous familial hypercholesterolemia (plaques of yellow color).

Fig. 2.16 Dermatofibroma sarcoma protuberans (nodule).

Fig. 2.17 Acute myelogenous leukemia (nodules).

Fig. 2.18 Erythema nodosum (subcutaneous nodules).

Fig. 2.19 Pyogenic granuloma (tumor). *Courtesy Curt Samlaska, MD.*

Fig. 2.20 Melanoma (tumor). *Courtesy Chris Miller, MD.*

Fig. 2.21 Basal cell carcinoma (tumor).

Fig. 2.22 Neurofibromatosis (macular hyperpigmentation, papules, tumors).

Fig. 2.23 Keloids (plaques and tumor).

Fig. 2.24 Acute urticaria (wheal). *Courtesy Curt Samlaska, MD.*

Fig. 2.25 Cold urticaria (wheal).

Fig. 2.28 Bullous pemphigoid (vesicles and bullae).

Fig. 2.26 Dyshidrosis (vesicles).

Fig. 2.29 Epidermolysis bullosa simplex (bullae). *Courtesy Scott Norton, MD.*

Fig. 2.27 Bullous pemphigoid (vesicles and bullae).

Fig. 2.30 Piroxicam hypersensitivity (vesicles and bullae, some with hemorrhage).

Fig. 2.31 Staphylococcal folliculitis (pustules).

Fig. 2.34 Staphylococcal folliculitis and impetigo (pustules and crusts).

Fig. 2.32 Plantar pustulosis (pustules).

Fig. 2.35 Hailey-Hailey disease (crusts).

Fig. 2.33 Autoinoculation vaccinia (umbillicated pustules).

Fig. 2.36 Paraneoplastic pemphigus (hemorrhagic crusts). *Courtesy Department of Dermatology, Keio University School of Medicine, Tokyo, Japan.*

Fig. 2.37 Chronic hand dermatitis from cement (scale).

Fig. 2.40 Congenital ichthyosiform erythroderma (scale with desquamation). *Courtesy Scott Norton, MD.*

Fig. 2.38 X-linked ichthyosis (scale).

Fig. 2.41 Toxic epidermal necrolysis (sheets of desquamation).

Fig. 2.39 Fogo selvagem (scale). *Courtesy Dermatology Division, University of Campinas, Brazil.*

Fig. 2.42 Morgellans disease (excoriations). *Courtesy Scott Norton, MD.*

Fig. 2.43 Chronic pruritus (linear excoriations).

Fig. 2.44 Perianal fissure (fissure).

Fig. 2.45 Bullous pemphigoid (erosion).

Fig. 2.46 Isotretinoin skin fragility in a college crew team member (erosions).

Fig. 2.47 Basal cell carcinoma (ulcer). *Courtesy Steven Binnick, MD.*

Fig. 2.48 Pyoderma gangrenosum (ulcer).

Fig. 2.49 Basal cell carcinoma (ulcer).

Fig. 2.52 Rounded scars and edema from skin popping.

Fig. 2.50 Atrophic scarring with milia in a patient with epidermolysis bullosa. *Courtesy Scott Norton, MD.*

Fig. 2.53 Keloid after voluntary branding. *Courtesy Scott Norton, MD.*

Fig. 2.51 Discoid lupus erythematosus (scarring alopecia). *Courtesy Steven Binnick, MD.*

Fig. 2.54 Keloid.

Fig. 2.55 Mycosis fungoides (poikiloderma). *Courtesy Steven Binnick, MD.*

Fig. 2.56 Limited scleroderma, CREST (gangrene).

Fig. 2.57 Atrophoderma (atrophy). *Courtesy Steven Binnick, MD.*

Fig. 2.58 Reeve sign (the reenactment of the cause of the condition during examination). Washboard nail dystrophy.

Fig. 2.59 Lichen simplex chronicus (lichenification).

Fig. 2.60 Lichen planus (linear, koebnerization).

Fig. 2.61 Granuloma annulare (annular).

Fig. 2.62 Tinea corporis (annular).

Fig. 2.63 Erythema ab igne (retiform).

Fig. 2.64 Cutaneous larva migrans (serpiginous).

Fig. 2.65 Herpes simplex (grouped).

Fig. 2.66 Linear epidermal nevus (blaschkoid).

Fig. 2.67 Systemic lupus erythematosus (photosensitivity pattern sparing nasolabial folds, under nose, under mouth). *Courtesy Steven Binnick, MD.*

Fig. 2.68 Melanoma (color variegation).

Fig. 2.69 Green nails from *Pseudomonas* infection (unusual color helps with the diagnosis).

Fig. 2.70 Pachyonychia congenita (oral).

Fig. 2.71 Kaposi sarcoma (conjunctiva).

Fig. 2.72 Nail groove from mucous cyst (nail).

Fig. 2.73 Alopecia areata (hair). *Courtesy Scott Norton, MD.*

Dermatoses Resulting from Physical Factors

3

This chapter catalogues many examples of how the skin reacts to the external environment from which it protects the body. Exposure to physical factors such as heat, cold, moisture, ultraviolet light, radiation, mechanical trauma and imbedded foreign bodies can manifest as uniquely patterned skin findings.

Of particular note are the many examples of photo-distributed eruptions, symmetrically involving the face, chest, dorsal hands and forearms, as this pattern can be an important physical exam clue to one of many specific photosensitive conditions. Those who spend significant amounts of time outdoors are particularly susceptible to acute and chronic sun damage and may also sustain temperature-related (cold or hot) injuries at acral sites.

The distribution of mechanical injuries and foreign body reactions, however, is usually asymmetric. In this chapter, appreciate the geometric shapes and unnatural configurations that can be produced on the skin as a result of physical abuse, radiotherapy or phytophotodermatitis. The patient history, and at times tissue analysis, can help to confirm the diagnosis that was suspected after a thorough physical examination.

This portion of the atlas features examples of dermatoses and skin lesions resulting from physical factors.

Fig. 3.1 Thermal burn from child abuse. *Courtesy Paul Honig, MD.*

Fig. 3.2 Hot water burn. *Courtesy Steven Binnick, MD.*

Fig. 3.3 Hot water bottle injury. *Courtesy Steven Binnick, MD.*

Fig. 3.4 Burn scar.

Fig. 3.5 Electrical burn from biting electrical cord. *Courtesy Paul Honig, MD.*

Fig. 3.6 Hot oil burn. *Courtesy Steven Binnick, MD.*

Fig. 3.7 Miliaria crystallina. *Courtesy Steven Binnick, MD.*

Fig. 3.8 Miliaria rubra.

Fig. 3.9 Miliaria rubra.

Fig. 3.10 Miliaria pustulosa secondary to childbirth. *Courtesy Curt Samlaska, MD.*

Fig. 3.11 Erythema ab igne. *Courtesy of Paul Honig, MD.*

Fig. 3.12 Erythema ab igne. *Courtesy of Misha Rosenbach, MD.*

Fig. 3.13 Pernio. *Courtesy Steven Binnick, MD.*

Fig. 3.14 Pernio.

Fig. 3.15 Pernio. *Courtesy Steven Binnick, MD.*

Fig. 3.16 Frostbite.

Fig. 3.17 Frostbite. *Courtesy Steven Binnick, MD.*

Fig. 3.18 Tropical immersion foot. *Courtesy Shyam Verma, MBBS, DVD.*

Fig. 3.19 Tropical immersion foot. *Courtesy Steven Binnick, MD.*

Fig. 3.20 Sunburn. *Courtesy Steven Binnick, MD.*

Fig. 3.21 Cutis rhomboidalis nuchae.

Fig. 3.22 Poikiloderma of Civatte.

Fig. 3.23 Favre-Racouchot.

Fig. 3.24 Favre-Racouchot with solar elastotic nodules.

Fig. 3.25 (A) Chronic solar damage. (B) With upward traction, normal non–sun-exposed skin is revealed.

Fig. 3.27 Solar elastosis of the forehead.

Fig. 3.26 Stellate pseudoscars.

Fig. 3.28 Weathering nodules.

Fig. 3.29 Colloid milium. *Courtesy Ken Greer, MD.*

Fig. 3.30 Photo onycholysis secondary to doxycycline. *Courtesy Lindsay Ackerman, MD.*

Fig. 3.31 Phytophotodermatitis.

Fig. 3.32 Two friends who made limeade in the sun to sell in the summer.

Fig. 3.33 Hyperpigmentation of the hand and cheek after phytophotodermatitis. *Courtesy Paul Honig, MD.*

Fig. 3.34 Polymorphous light eruption, papular type.

Fig. 3.35 Polymorphous light eruption, papular type.

Fig. 3.36 Polymorphous light eruption, plaque type.

Fig. 3.37 Juvenile spring eruption of the ears.

Fig. 3.38 Actinic prurigo. *Courtesy Steven Binnick, MD.*

Fig. 3.39 Actinic prurigo. *Courtesy Campbell Stewart, MD.*

Fig. 3.40 Solar urticaria.

Fig. 3.41 Hydroa vacciniforme. *Courtesy Paul Honig, MD.*

Fig. 3.42 Chronic actinic dermatitis.

Fig. 3.43 Chronic actinic dermatitis.

Fig. 3.44 Chronic radiodermatitis.

Fig. 3.45 Chronic radiodermatitis with fibrosis. *Courtesy Steven Binnick, MD.*

Fig. 3.46 Chronic radiodermatitis with basal cell cancer as a complication. *Courtesy Steven Binnick, MD.*

Fig. 3.47 (A) Fluoroscopy-induced radiodermatitis. (B) Close-up of Fig. 3.47A.

Fig. 3.48 Hard corn. *Courtesy Steven Binnick, MD.*

Fig. 3.49 Soft corn. *Courtesy Steven Binnick, MD.*

Fig. 3.50 Fire coral cuts. *Courtesy Steven Binnick, MD.*

Fig. 3.51 Decubitus ulcer. *Courtesy Steven Binnick, MD.*

Fig. 3.52 Sclerosing lymphangitis.

Fig. 3.53 (A) Black heel. (B) Immediately after scraping off blood from black heel.

Fig. 3.54 Subcutaneous emphysema. *Courtesy Curt Samlaska, MD.*

Fig. 3.55 Piezogenic papules. *Courtesy Paul Honig, MD.*

Fig. 3.56 Skin-popping ulcer.

Fig. 3.57 Cotton granuloma.

Fig. 3.58 Hair granuloma in a barber.

Fig. 3.59 Red tattoo reaction. *Courtesy Rui Tavares Bello, MD.*

Fig. 3.60 Silicone granuloma.

Fig. 3.61 Mercury granuloma from thermometer.

Fig. 3.62 Silica granuloma.

Fig. 3.63 Carbon stain, gunshot wound.

Fig. 3.64 Zyplast granuloma, test site.

Pruritus and Neurocutaneous Diseases

Pruritus often produces distinctive skin lesions, characterized by angulated borders. Endogenous diseases (in common parlance, an "inside job") tend to produce lesions that are rounded in character, whereas exogenous caustic agents, scratching, and other forms of external trauma tend to produce angulated, linear, or geometric shapes (signs of an "outside job").

Pruritus can also result in the isomorphic (Koebner) phenomenon, where lesions of an endogenous disease localize in areas of trauma. These lesions often demonstrate a hybrid morphology, suggesting both endogenous origin and external trauma.

Lichenification results from chronic scratching or rubbing and is characterized by hyperkeratosis and papillary dermal fibrosis. The resulting clinical morphology includes slight induration and accentuation of skin markings. Excoriation results in eosinophilic necrosis of the granular layer. The corneum can remain intact, but more severe excoriation results in loss of the corneum and viable epidermis. More pronounced trauma can result in ulceration, in which the injury extends to the level of the dermis.

Broad areas of lichenification are characteristic of lichen simplex chronicus. Discrete papules with focal evidence of excoriation are typical of prurigo nodularis and arthropod bites, including those caused by bedbugs. This portion of the atlas will guide you through the clinical manifestations related to pruritic disorders.

Fig. 4.2 Acquired perforating disease in renal failure.

Fig. 4.1 Excoriations secondary to pruritus of Hodgkin disease.

Fig. 4.3 Acquired perforating disease in renal failure.

Fig. 4.4 Acquired perforating disease in renal failure. *Courtesy Steven Binnick, MD.*

Fig. 4.5 Prurigo nodularis in a chronic renal failure patient. *Courtesy Steven Binnick, MD.*

Fig. 4.6 Jaundice.

Fig. 4.7 Palmar xanthomas in hepatic cholestasis.

Fig. 4.8 Lichen simplex chronicus in Alagille disease.

Fig. 4.9 Hyperpigmentation in primary biliary cirrhosis.

Fig. 4.10 Winter itch.

Fig. 4.11 Lichen simplex chronicus in pruritus ani.

Fig. 4.12 Lichen simplex chronicus of the scrotum.

Fig. 4.13 Lichen simplex chronicus of the vulva.

Fig. 4.14 Prurigo pigmentosa.

Fig. 4.15 Prurigo pigmentosa. *Courtesy Stephen D. Hess, MD, PhD.*

Fig. 4.16 Prurigo pigmentosa. *Courtesy of Department of Dermatology, Keio University School of Medicine, Tokyo, Japan.*

Fig. 4.17 Papuloerythroderma of Ofuji with deck chair sign. *Courtesy Dr. Ang Chia Chun.*

Fig. 4.18 Lichen simplex chronicus.

Fig. 4.19 Lichen simplex chronicus.

Fig. 4.20 Lichen simplex chronicus.

Fig. 4.21 Lichen simplex chronicus. *Courtesy Steven Binnick, MD.*

Fig. 4.22 Lichen simplex chronicus with dyspigmentation and early nodule formation.

Fig. 4.23 Prurigo nodularis.

Fig. 4.24 Prurigo nodularis with excoriation.

Fig. 4.25 Compulsive finger biting.

Fig. 4.26 Chronic lip licking. *Courtesy Steven Binnick, MD.*

Fig. 4.27 Dryness secondary to compulsive hand washing.

Fig. 4.28 Washboard nails secondary to habitual trauma to the matrix.

Fig. 4.29 Fibroma secondary to chronic tongue biting. *Courtesy of the Department of Oral Medicine, the University of Pennsylvania School of Dental Medicine.*

Fig. 4.30 Enamel erosion secondary to vomiting with bulimia. *Courtesy of the Department of Oral Medicine, the University of Pennsylvania School of Dental Medicine.*

Fig. 4.31 Delusions of parasitosis.

Fig. 4.32 Delusions of parasitosis.

Fig. 4.33 Psychogenic excoriations. *Courtesy Steven Binnick, MD.*

Fig. 4.34 Psychogenic excoriations. *Courtesy Curt Samlaska, MD.*

Fig. 4.35 Skin picking in Prader-Willi syndrome. *Courtesy Robert Horn, MD.*

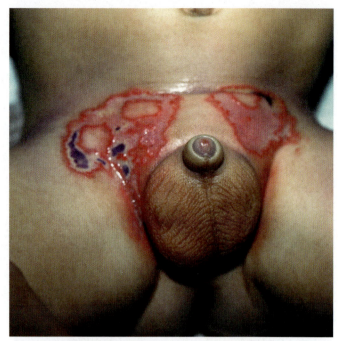

Fig. 4.36 Factitial ulcers induced by parents.

Fig. 4.37 Factitial dermatitis.

Fig. 4.38 Factitial ulcers.

Fig. 4.39 Cigarette burn, factitial.

Fig. 4.40 Factitial ulcer.

Fig. 4.41 Factitial bruising.

Fig. 4.42 Factitial blisters and erosions. *Courtesy Steven Binnick, MD.*

Fig. 4.43 Factitial scarring.

Fig. 4.44 Healed factitial lacerations. *Courtesy Sheilagh Maguiness, MD.*

Fig. 4.45 Factitial ulcers and scarring.

Fig. 4.46 Factitial erosions and scarring.

Fig. 4.47 Trichotillosis, with loss of eyelashes and partial loss of eyebrows. *Courtesy Steven Binnick, MD.*

Fig. 4.48 Trichotillosis, with partial loss of eyelashes. *Courtesy Steven Binnick, MD.*

Fig. 4.49 Trichotillosis.

Fig. 4.50 Notalgia paresthetica. *Courtesy Curt Samlaska, MD.*

Fig. 4.51 Complex regional pain syndrome.

Fig. 4.52 Complex regional pain syndrome.

Fig. 4.53 Blistering and atrophy, complex regional pain syndrome.

Fig. 4.54 Trigeminal trophic syndrome. *Courtesy Division of Dermatology University of Campinas, Brazil.*

Fig. 4.55 Neuropathic ulcer of the hand in a diabetic patient.

Atopic Dermatitis, Eczema, and Noninfectious Immunodeficiency Disorders

Dermatitis can present with a variety of physical examination findings ranging from exuberant oozing to dry scale. These findings represent the acute and chronic inflammation that defines a variety of dermatitides and eczematous conditions. Intense itching that accompanies these conditions can lead to overlying excoriations and eventually thickening of the skin known as *lichenification*. Ultimately, constant itching and a poor epidermal barrier predispose patients with these eczematous conditions to repeated skin infections from bacteria and viruses, which can present with pustules, vesicles, crusting, erosions, or painful nodules. Screening for signs of such infections is an important part of the physical examination for all patients with dermatitis, especially those with any underlying immunodeficiency.

Although most cases will not require a skin biopsy for a diagnosis, the spongiosis of acute dermatitis or the acanthosis of the epidermis seen in chronic dermatitis can be confirmatory in scenarios wherein other diagnoses that affect the epidermis are being considered, such as nutritional deficiencies, graft-versus-host disease, or psoriasis.

The anatomic location of atopic dermatitis (AD) can vary depending on age. Infantile AD tends to affect the cheeks and can have impressive overlying exudation and crusting even in the absence of infection. In infants, AD can also be quite widespread with predilections for extensor surfaces and notable sparing of the diaper region and nose, the so-called *headlight sign*. Childhood AD may be more localized to the flexors and can begin to take on a more lichenified appearance. Many people with AD will outgrow a more widespread dermatitis, but may have chronic hand dermatitis or other more localized flares of their AD. Associated features of AD found on physical examination include Dennie-Morgan lines (accentuated folds of the lower eyelids), keratosis pilaris, general xerosis, follicular accentuation, and signs of atopy such as hyperpigmentation around the eyes known as *allergic shiners*.

Other forms of eczema may take on different patterns on the body, including the coin-shaped, scaly, and exudative plaques of nummular eczema or the diffuse, dry, and cracked appearance of xerotic eczema (eczema craquele). Even in patients without a history of AD, localized forms of eczema may arise on the eyelids or nipples, or on the hands as vesiculobullous hand eczema (pompholyx). Finally, some forms of immunodeficiency disorders can present with relatively nonspecific exfoliative erythroderma, as in severe combined immunodeficiency (SCID), or an atopic dermatitis-like eruption, as in hyper–immunoglobulinemia E (IgE) syndrome, Wiskott-Aldrich syndrome (WAS), or DiGeorge syndrome. In these cases, the astute clinician will observe distinctive clinical findings such as the pustular eruption of hyper-IgE syndrome, dysmorphisms of DiGeorge syndrome, or petechiae within the dermatitis of patients with WAS. This portion of the atlas will highlight the range of clinical findings seen in patients with atopic dermatitis and other forms of eczema, along with rarer findings seen in patients with immunodeficiency syndromes.

Fig. 5.1 Atopic dermatitis.

Fig. 5.2 Atopic dermatitis.

Fig. 5.3 Atopic dermatitis.

Fig. 5.4 Chronic atopic dermatitis.

Fig. 5.5 Atopic dermatitis with excoriations.

Fig. 5.6 Atopic dermatitis with secondary infection. *Courtesy Steven Binnick, MD.*

Fig. 5.7 Atopic dermatitis.

Fig. 5.8 Atopic dermatitis.

Fig. 5.9 Atopic dermatitis with secondary infection.

Fig. 5.10 Atopic dermatitis.

Fig. 5.11 Chronic atopic dermatitis.

Fig. 5.12 Chronic atopic dermatitis.

Fig. 5.13 Chronic atopic dermatitis with hyperpigmentation.

Fig. 5.14 Atopic dermatitis, lichenification. *Courtesy Steven Binnick, MD.*

Fig. 5.15 Atopic dermatitis. *Courtesy Steven Binnick, MD.*

Fig. 5.16 Papular atopic dermatitis. *Courtesy Steven Binnick, MD.*

Fig. 5.17 Atopic dermatitis. *Courtesy Steven Binnick, MD.*

Fig. 5.18 Atopic dermatitis with Dennie-Morgan lines. *Courtesy Steven Binnick, MD.*

Fig. 5.19 White dermatographism.

Fig. 5.20 Erythroderma from atopic dermatitis.

Fig. 5.21 Pityriasis alba. *Courtesy Steven Binnick, MD.*

Fig. 5.22 Hyperlinear palms in a patient with active atopic dermatitis. *Courtesy Steven Binnick, MD.*

Fig. 5.23 Keratosis pilaris. *Courtesy Steven Binnick, MD.*

Fig. 5.24 Keratosis pilaris.

Fig. 5.25 Keratosis pilaris rubra faciei.

Fig. 5.26 Eczema herpeticum. *Courtesy Paul Honig, MD.*

Fig. 5.27 Ear eczema.

Fig. 5.28 Eyelid eczema.

Fig. 5.29 Nipple eczema in an atopic child.

Fig. 5.30 Hand dermatitis with secondary infection.

Fig. 5.31 Finger dermatitis from primrose allergy.

Fig. 5.32 Pompholyx.

Fig. 5.33 Pompholyx.

Fig. 5.34 Irritant diaper dermatitis. Note sparing of folds.

Fig. 5.35 Id reaction.

Fig. 5.36 Xerotic eczema.

Fig. 5.37 Nummular eczema.

Fig. 5.38 Nummular eczema. *Courtesy Steven Binnick, MD.*

Fig. 5.39 Job's syndrome. *Courtesy Edward W. Cowen, MD.*

Fig. 5.40 Job's syndrome. *Courtesy Edward W. Cowen, MD.*

Fig. 5.41 Job's syndrome with secondary infection. *Courtesy Paul Honig, MD.*

Fig. 5.42 Eczema in Wiskott-Aldrich syndrome.

Fig. 5.43 Ataxia telangiectasia.

Fig. 5.44 Granulomatous lesions in ataxia telangiectasia.

Fig. 5.45 Common variable immunodeficiency with granulomas in vitiligo.

Fig. 5.46 Common variable immunodeficiency with granulomas in vitiligo.

Fig. 5.47 Common variable immunodeficiency with chronic candidiasis.

Fig. 5.48 Warts in DOCK8 immunodeficiency. *Courtesy Edward W. Cowen, MD.*

Fig. 5.49 Warts in DOCK8 immunodeficiency. *Courtesy Edward W. Cowen, MD.*

Fig. 5.50 Warts in DOCK8 immunodeficiency. *Courtesy Edward W. Cowen, MD.*

Fig. 5.51 Subacute lupus erythematosus as can be seen in complement deficiency disorders.

Fig. 5.52 Acute graft-versus-host disease.

Fig. 5.53 Acute graft-versus-host disease grade 2. *Courtesy Jennifer Huang, MD.*

Fig. 5.54 Acute graft-versus-host disease grade 2. *Courtesy Jennifer Huang, MD.*

Fig. 5.55 Acute graft-versus-host disease grade 4. *Courtesy Jennifer Huang, MD.*

Fig. 5.56 Acute graft-versus-host disease. *Courtesy Edward W. Cowen, MD.*

Fig. 5.57 Lichenoid graft-versus-host disease. *Courtesy Jennifer Huang, MD.*

Fig. 5.58 Chronic graft-versus-host disease. *Courtesy Jennifer Huang, MD.*

Fig. 5.59 Chronic graft-versus-host disease, oral. *Courtesy of the Department of Oral Medicine, the University of Pennsylvania School of Dental Medicine.*

Fig. 5.60 Chronic graft-versus-host disease, sclerodermoid type. *Courtesy Edward W. Cowen, MD.*

Fig. 5.61 Chronic graft-versus-host disease. *Courtesy Edward W. Cowen, MD.*

Fig. 5.62 Sclerodermoid graft-versus-host disease. *Courtesy Edward W. Cowen, MD.*

Fig. 5.63 Sclerodermoid graft-versus-host disease. *Courtesy Edward W. Cowen, MD.*

Fig. 5.64 Fasciitis in graft-versus-host disease. *Courtesy Edward W. Cowen, MD.*

Contact Dermatitis and Drug Eruptions

Contact dermatitis and cutaneous drug eruptions are both skin conditions triggered by external agents that are either in direct contact with the skin or ingested. Contact dermatitis shares many features with atopic dermatitis and eczema, including pruritus, erythema, scaling, oozing, and crusting. However, in the case of contact dermatitis, major clues to the diagnosis are the shapes found on the skin that demonstrate the particular locations of contact by the external irritant or allergic stimuli. These shapes can be classically *linear* like *Toxicodendron dermatitis* (poison ivy); *geometric* such as seen secondary to adhesives; in a *splattered pattern* secondary to liquid irritants (e.g., acids); or in the case of airborne triggers such as fragrances, concentrated on the face, neck, and other exposed regions of the body. Noting the location of the affected body part or parts is especially helpful in diagnosing contact dermatitis, such as the lower abdomen and ears in nickel dermatitis, dorsal feet in shoe dermatitis, and eyelids in dermatitis secondary to ingredients in nail polish. Other contact reactions can be more widespread, as is the case in some patients with atopic dermatitis and concomitant contact dermatitis due to preservatives or fragrances in lotions and detergents, respectively.

Cutaneous drug eruptions can be quite varied in their presentations, ranging from the sheets of micropustules overlying patches of broad erythema seen in acute generalized exanthematous pustulosis to the hemorrhagic mucosal erosions and vesicobullous lesions seen in Stevens-Johnson syndrome and toxic epidermal necrolysis. It is imperative to screen patients for associated features on physical examination such as fever, lymphadenopathy, and facial edema that can help distinguish a systemic drug hypersensitivity reaction such as drug reaction with eosinophilia and systemic symptoms (DRESS) from a simple morbilliform drug eruption. Blood work may also be needed in some patients with suspected DRESS to screen for eosinophilia, atypical lymphocytes, and evidence of end organ damage. Other drug eruptions may be more unique, such as the striking, deeply erythematous, circular patches and plaques of fixed drug eruptions or painful palmoplantar plaques of toxic erythema of chemotherapy. Because new medications are being produced every year, it is also important to remain knowledgeable about the diverse idiosyncratic drug eruptions such as the erosive psoriasiform scalp and posterior auricular plaques seen in individuals treated with tumor necrosis factor inhibitors.

This portion of the atlas will highlight the cutaneous patterns created by contact dermatitis, as well as the variety of skin findings seen in the setting of both mild and severe drug eruptions.

Fig. 6.1 Cement burns. *Courtesy Steven Binnick, MD.*

Fig. 6.2 Acid burn. *Courtesy Paul Honig, MD.*

Fig. 6.3 Drip burn from acid solution.

Fig. 6.4 Senna burn.

Fig. 6.5 Pesticide burn.

Fig. 6.6 Irritant dermatitis from kerosene. *Courtesy Shyam Verma, MBBS, DVD.*

Fig. 6.7 Positive patch test.

Fig. 6.8 Poison ivy dermatitis; note linear lesions.

Fig. 6.9 Poison ivy dermatitis; note linear lesions.

Fig. 6.10 Poison ivy dermatitis.

Fig. 6.11 Poison ivy dermatitis.

Fig. 6.12 Poison ivy dermatitis.

Fig. 6.13 Tea tree oil dermatitis. *Courtesy Glen Crawford, MD.*

Fig. 6.14 Clothing contact dermatitis.

Fig. 6.15 (A) Blue dye dermatitis. (B) Resolved when using diapers without blue dye.

Fig. 6.16 Acute shoe dermatitis.

Fig. 6.17 Chronic shoe dermatitis. *Courtesy of Steven Binnick, MD.*

Fig. 6.18 (A) Nickel dermatitis. (B) With earrings on.

Fig. 6.19 Nickel dermatitis.

Fig. 6.20 Black dermatographism. *Courtesy Steven Binnick, MD.*

Fig. 6.21 Oral lichenoid dermatitis due to gold.

Fig. 6.22 Stomatitis due to dental impression material allergy.

Fig. 6.23 (A) Rubber dermatitis. (B) Culprit swim goggles.

Fig. 6.24 Earbud dermatitis.

Fig. 6.25 Contact allergy to adhesive in bandage.

Fig. 6.26 Hand dermatitis due to aromatherapy. *Courtesy Glen Crawford, MD.*

Fig. 6.27 Eyelid dermatitis secondary to nail polish.

Fig. 6.28 Hair dye dermatitis. *Courtesy Steven Binnick, MD.*

Fig. 6.29 Vulvar dermatitis secondary to preservatives.

Fig. 6.30 Clonidine patch allergy.

Fig. 6.31 Allergy to benzocaine.

Fig. 6.32 Allergy to topical antibiotic.

Fig. 6.33 Leg ulcer with contact dermatitis due to topical antibiotic allergy.

Fig. 6.34 Contact allergy to topical steroids.

Fig. 6.35 Contact cheilitis to Blistik.

Fig. 6.36 Contact dermatitis to eye drops. *Courtesy Shyam Verma, MBBS, DVD.*

Fig. 6.37 Contact urticaria to surgical gloves. *Courtesy Arto Lahti, MD.*

Fig. 6.38 Drug eruption.

Fig. 6.39 Drug eruption.

Fig. 6.40 (A) Drug eruption in leukemic patient. (B) Drug eruption in leukemic patient with low platelet count. The exanthem may be purpuric.

Fig. 6.41 Phenytoin-induced drug reaction with eosinophilia and systemic symptoms.

Fig. 6.42 Phenytoin-induced drug reaction with eosinophilia and systemic symptoms.

Fig. 6.43 Phenytoin-induced drug reaction with eosinophilia and systemic symptoms.

Fig. 6.44 Stevens-Johnson syndrome secondary to *Mycoplasma* infection.

Fig. 6.45 Stevens-Johnson syndrome.

Fig. 6.46 Stevens-Johnson syndrome. *Courtesy Steven Binnick, MD.*

Fig. 6.47 Phenytoin-induced Stevens-Johnson syndrome.

Fig. 6.48 Toxic epidermal necrolysis to Lamotrigine.

Fig. 6.49 Toxic epidermal necrolysis to Lamotrigine.

Fig. 6.50 Toxic epidermal necrolysis.

Fig. 6.51 Phenytoin plus radiation-induced reaction.

Fig. 6.52 Sulfa allergy in an HIV-infected patient.

Fig. 6.53 Fixed drug reaction. *Courtesy Steven Binnick, MD.*

Fig. 6.54 Fixed drug reaction on lower lip.

Fig. 6.55 Fixed drug reaction.

Fig. 6.56 Fixed drug reaction.

Fig. 6.57 Fixed drug reaction. *Courtesy Steven Binnick, MD.*

Fig. 6.58 Acute generalized exanthematous pustulosis.

Fig. 6.59 Acute generalized exanthematous pustulosis.

Fig. 6.60 Acute generalized exanthematous pustulosis. *Courtesy Sheilagh Maguiness, MD.*

Fig. 6.61 Acute generalized exanthematous pustulosis. *Courtesy Sheilagh Maguiness, MD.*

Fig. 6.62 Urticaria. *Courtesy Steven Binnick, MD.*

Fig. 6.63 Voriconazole phototoxicity. *Courtesy Jennifer Huang, MD.*

Fig. 6.64 Voriconazole phototoxicity. *Courtesy Edward W. Cowen, MD.*

Fig. 6.65 Minocycline-induced photosensitivity.

Fig. 6.66 Piroxicam photosensitivity.

Fig. 6.67 Photosensitivity to quinine.

Fig. 6.68 Quinidine photo-induced livedo reticularis.

Fig. 6.69 Warfarin-induced necrosis. *Courtesy Steven Binnick, MD.*

Fig. 6.70 Warfarin-induced necrosis. *Courtesy Steven Binnick, MD.*

Fig. 6.71 Vitamin K injection site reaction.

Fig. 6.72 Vitamin K injection site reaction.

Fig. 6.73 Intravenous extravasation with necrosis.

Fig. 6.74 Amiodarone hyperpigmentation.

Fig. 6.75 Doxorubicin hyperpigmentation.

Fig. 6.76 Chrysiasis.

Fig. 6.77 Chlorpromazine hyperpigmentation.

Fig. 6.78 Minocycline hyperpigmentation.

Fig. 6.79 Minocycline hyperpigmentation.

Fig. 6.80 Minocycline hyperpigmentation.

Fig. 6.81 Minocycline hyperpigmentation.

Fig. 6.82 Minocycline hyperpigmentation.

Fig. 6.83 Doxorubicin hyperpigmentation.

Fig. 6.84 Chemotherapy-induced transverse nail hyperpigmentation.

Fig. 6.85 Chloroquine hyperpigmentation.

Fig. 6.86 Methotrexate-induced vascular hyperpigmentation. *Courtesy Steven Binnick, MD.*

Fig. 6.87 Bleomycin flagellate hyperpigmentation.

Fig. 6.88 Serum sickness–like reaction.

Fig. 6.89 Lichenoid drug reaction.

Fig. 6.90 Lichenoid drug reaction.

Fig. 6.91 Methotrexate-induced oral ulcers.

Fig. 6.92 Radiation recall induced by vemurafenib.

Fig. 6.93 Toxic erythema of chemotherapy.

Fig. 6.94 Toxic erythema of chemotherapy.

Fig. 6.95 Neutrophilic eccrine hidradenitis. *Courtesy Misha Rosenbach, MD.*

Fig. 6.96 Neutrophilic eccrine hidradenitis. *Courtesy Robert Micheletti, MD.*

Fig. 6.97 Pembrolizumab-associated vitiligo.

Fig. 6.98 BRAF inhibitor–induced hand-foot reaction. *Courtesy Emily Chu, MD, PhD.*

Fig. 6.99 Tumor necrosis factor inhibitor–related psoriasiform reaction.

Fig. 6.100 Epidermal growth factor inhibitor–induced acneiform reaction.

Fig. 6.101 Epidermal growth factor inhibitor–induced paronychia.

Fig. 6.102 Granulocyte colony stimulating factor reaction.

Fig. 6.103 Pink disease (mercury toxicity).

Fig. 6.104 Follicular iododerma.

Fig. 6.105 Topical steroid–induced atrophy. *Courtesy Steven Binnick, MD.*

Fig. 6.106 Topical steroid–induced atrophy. *Courtesy Steven Binnick, MD.*

Fig. 6.107 Lipoatrophy after steroid injection. *Courtesy Steven Binnick, MD.*

Fig. 6.108 Hypopigmentation after intralesional steroid injection.

Erythema and Urticaria

A wide variety of conditions can present with erythema or urticarial lesions. Whereas many conditions such as urticaria and angioedema lack identifiable surface changes, other diagnoses in this chapter have distinctive scaling. Pustules and ulcerations are seen in some cases as a manifestation of intense underlying, often neutrophilic, inflammation.

Many of the erythemas in this portion of the atlas share an annular and polycyclic morphology, including urticaria, erythema annulare centrifugum, and erythema gyratum repens, but only erythema multiforme demonstrates the true fixed target lesion. Noting whether skin findings are migratory or fixed is helpful in distinguishing common urticaria from many other more fixed lesions. Skin testing to demonstrate dermatographism is also helpful as a bedside technique to recapitulate urticaria in a susceptible patient. Ultimately, a skin biopsy may be needed to differentiate reactive neutrophilic dermatoses, such as Sweet syndrome (acute febrile neutrophilic dermatosis), from eosinophilic conditions, such as Wells syndrome (eosinophilic cellulitis). Tissue cultures are often needed when diagnosing pyoderma gangrenosum to rule out infectious etiologies such as bacteria, fungi, or atypical mycobacteria, depending on the clinical setting.

This portion of the atlas features examples of urticaria, urticarial lesions, erythemas, and angioedema.

Fig. 7.1 Flushing.

Fig. 7.2 Palmar erythema.

Fig. 7.3 Erythema toxicum neonatorum.

Fig. 7.4 Erythema toxicum neonatorum.

Fig. 7.6 Erythema multiforme. *Courtesy Steven Binnick, MD.*

Fig. 7.5 Erythema multiforme. *Courtesy Steven Binnick, MD.*

Fig. 7.7 Erythema multiforme secondary to sulfa.

Fig. 7.8 Erythema multiforme. *Courtesy Steven Binnick, MD.*

Fig. 7.9 Erythema multiforme.

Fig. 7.10 Erythema multiforme.

Fig. 7.11 Erythema multiforme. *Courtesy Steven Binnick, MD.*

Fig. 7.12 Erythema multiforme. *Courtesy Steven Binnick, MD.*

Fig. 7.13 Erythema multiforme.

Fig. 7.14 Stevens-Johnson syndrome.

Fig. 7.15 Toxic epidermal necrolysis.

Fig. 7.16 Urticaria multiforme.

Fig. 7.17 Urticaria multiforme.

Fig. 7.18 Recurrent oral erythema multiforme.

Fig. 7.19 Recurrent oral erythema multiforme.

Fig. 7.20 Recurrent oral erythema multiforme. *Courtesy Steven Binnick, MD.*

Fig. 7.21 Erythema annulare centrifugum.

Fig. 7.22 Erythema annulare centrifugum.

Fig. 7.23 Erythema annulare centrifugum.

Fig. 7.24 Erythema gyratum repens. *Courtesy Donald Lookingbill, MD.*

Fig. 7.25 Eosinophilic annular erythema.

Fig. 7.26 Wells syndrome. *Courtesy Glen Crawford, MD.*

Fig. 7.27 Sweet syndrome.

Fig. 7.28 Sweet syndrome with acute myelogenous leukemia.

Fig. 7.29 Sweet syndrome.

Fig. 7.30 Sweet syndrome.

Fig. 7.31 Sweet syndrome.

Fig. 7.32 Sweet syndrome.

Fig. 7.33 Sweet syndrome in a patient with systemic lupus erythematosus.

Fig. 7.34 Sweet syndrome in acute myelogenous leukemia.

Fig. 7.35 Sweet syndrome in leukemia. *Courtesy Misha Rosenbach, MD.*

Fig. 7.36 Sweet syndrome in acute leukemia.

Fig. 7.37 Sweet syndrome.

Fig. 7.38 Histiocytoid Sweet syndrome. *Courtesy Misha Rosenbach, MD.*

Fig. 7.39 Lymphocytic Sweet syndrome.

Fig. 7.40 Neutrophilic dermatosis of the dorsal hands.

Fig. 7.41 Neutrophilic dermatosis of the dorsal hands.

Fig. 7.42 Neutrophilic dermatosis of the dorsal hands.

Fig. 7.43 Early pyoderma gangrenosum.

Fig. 7.44 Pyoderma gangrenosum. *Courtesy Steven Binnick, MD.*

Fig. 7.45 Pyoderma gangrenosum. *Courtesy Misha Rosenbach, MD.*

Fig. 7.46 Pyoderma gangrenosum. *Courtesy Paul Honig, MD.*

Fig. 7.47 Pyoderma gangrenosum in an HIV-infected patient. *Courtesy Steven Binnick, MD.*

Fig. 7.48 Healing pyoderma gangrenosum. *Courtesy of Curt Samlaska, MD.*

Fig. 7.49 Cryopyrin-associated periodic fever syndrome with Muckle-Wells syndrome. *Courtesy Karoline Krause, MD.*

Fig. 7.50 Cryopyrin-associated periodic syndrome with atypical pernio-like lesions.

Fig. 7.51 Schnitzler syndrome. *Courtesy Karoline Krause, MD.*

Fig. 7.52 Urticaria.

Fig. 7.53 Urticaria. *Courtesy Steven Binnick, MD.*

Fig. 7.54 Urticaria. *Courtesy Steven Binnick, MD.*

Fig. 7.55 Urticaria.

Fig. 7.56 Cold urticaria. *Courtesy Steven Binnick, MD.*

Fig. 7.57 Cold urticaria.

Fig. 7.58 Cold urticaria.

Fig. 7.59 Exercise-induced urticaria.

Fig. 7.60 Cholinergic urticaria.

Fig. 7.61 Cholinergic urticaria.

Fig. 7.62 Cholinergic urticaria.

Fig. 7.63 Solar urticaria.

Fig. 7.64 Delayed pressure urticaria.

Fig. 7.65 Dermatographism.

Fig. 7.66 Dermatographism. *Courtesy Curt Samlaska, MD.*

Fig. 7.67 Dermatographism.

Fig. 7.68 Angioedema.

Fig. 7.69 Angioedema. *Courtesy Steven Binnick, MD.*

Connective Tissue Diseases

Cutaneous manifestations of connective tissue diseases are important to identify because they can be a clue to an undiagnosed systemic autoimmune disease. Many lesions, such as those seen in systemic lupus erythematosus (SLE) and dermatomyositis (DM), share a notable bright pink or purplish color, likely due to the intense lymphocytic inflammation found at the dermal-epidermal junction. Photosensitivity, as demonstrated best by the malar erythema of SLE and DM, is another shared feature of some connective tissue diseases, and therefore recognizing a photodistributed pattern is again important in this portion of the atlas.

Each subtype of lupus erythematosus has notable physical examination findings, including the scarring and dyspigmentation seen in discoid lupus erythematosus, the annular psoriasiform plaques of subacute cutaneous lupus erythematosus and neonatal lupus erythematosus, and the deeper palpable nodules or depressions of lupus profundus. Classically seen in DM as the heliotrope sign, some patients with DM or SLE will present with purplish patches of the eyelids.

This chapter also includes the spectrum of skin findings seen in localized and systemic scleroderma. Localized scleroderma (morphea) presents with an expanding, indurated, pink or lilac sometimes circinate, plaque that leaves scarlike dyspigmentation centrally and can lead to disfigurement, joint contractures, and skin ulcerations. In contrast, limited and systemic scleroderma present with distinctive cutaneous signs such as matlike telangiectasias, calcinosis cutis, and, in some, a symmetric, progressive, woody edema.

Patients with suspected connective tissue disease deserve a full review of systems and physical examination for rarer mucocutaneous findings, such as mucosal erosions or ulcerations, alopecia, sclerodactyly, nailfold capillary changes, and lymphadenopathy. Skin biopsies are almost always warranted and helpful when gathering information to confirm some of these difficult diagnoses.

This portion of the atlas features the aforementioned and other rarer connective tissue diseases and their multitude of cutaneous stigmata.

Fig. 8.1 Discoid lupus erythematosus.

Fig. 8.2 Discoid lupus erythematosus.

Fig. 8.3 Discoid lupus erythematosus. *Courtesy Steven Binnick, MD.*

Fig. 8.4 Discoid lupus erythematosus. *Courtesy Steven Binnick, MD.*

Fig. 8.5 Discoid lupus erythematosus.

Fig. 8.6 Discoid lupus erythematosus. *Courtesy Steven Binnick, MD.*

Fig. 8.7 Discoid lupus erythematosus.

Fig. 8.8 Discoid lupus erythematosus.

Fig. 8.9 Discoid lupus erythematosus. *Courtesy Steven Binnick, MD.*

Fig. 8.10 Discoid lupus erythematosus. *Courtesy Steven Binnick, MD.*

Fig. 8.11 Generalized discoid lupus erythematosus. *Courtesy Steven Binnick, MD.*

Fig. 8.12 Generalized discoid lupus erythematosus. *Courtesy Steven Binnick, MD.*

Fig. 8.13 Hypertrophic lupus erythematosus. *Courtesy Steven Binnick, MD.*

Fig. 8.14 Hypertrophic lupus erythematosus. *Courtesy Steven Binnick, MD.*

Fig. 8.15 Lichen planus lupus erythematosus overlap. *Courtesy Ken Greer, MD.*

Fig. 8.16 Lupus profundus.

Fig. 8.17 Lupus profundus.

Fig. 8.18 Lupus profundus. *Courtesy Curt Samlaska, MD.*

Fig. 8.19 Lupus profundus with resultant atrophy.

Fig. 8.20 Tumid lupus erythematosus.

Fig. 8.21 Tumid lupus erythematosus.

Fig. 8.22 Subacute cutaneous lupus erythematosus. *Courtesy Steven Binnick, MD.*

Fig. 8.23 Subacute cutaneous lupus erythematosus.

Fig. 8.24 Subacute cutaneous lupus erythematosus.

Fig. 8.25 Subacute cutaneous lupus erythematosus.

Fig. 8.26 Neonatal lupus erythematosus.

Fig. 8.27 Neonatal lupus erythematosus with scarring.

Fig. 8.28 Neonatal lupus erythematosus.

Fig. 8.29 Neonatal lupus erythematosus.

Fig. 8.30 Acute systemic lupus erythematosus.

Fig. 8.31 Acute systemic lupus erythematosus.

Fig. 8.32 Acute systemic lupus erythematosus. *Courtesy Paul Honig, MD.*

Fig. 8.33 Acute systemic lupus erythematosus.

Fig. 8.34 Systemic lupus erythematosus with dyspigmentation. Note sparing over the proximal interphalangeal and metacarpophalangeal joints.

Fig. 8.35 Alopecia in systemic lupus erythematosus.

Fig. 8.36 Systemic lupus erythematosus.

Fig. 8.37 Chilblain systemic lupus erythematosus with painful scars.

Fig. 8.38 Bullous systemic lupus erythematosus.

Fig. 8.39 Bullous systemic lupus erythematosus.

Fig. 8.40 Palisaded neutrophilic granulomatous dermatitis.

Fig. 8.41 Palisaded neutrophilic granulomatous dermatitis.

Fig. 8.42 Palisaded neutrophilic granulomatous dermatitis.

Fig. 8.43 Oral lupus erythematosus.

Fig. 8.44 Oral lupus erythematosus.

Fig. 8.45 Oral lupus erythematosus.

Fig. 8.46 Skin lesions secondary to antiphospholipid antibodies in systemic lupus erythematosus.

Fig. 8.47 Skin lesions secondary to antiphospholipid antibodies in systemic lupus erythematosus.

Fig. 8.48 Dermatomyositis, heliotrope.

Fig. 8.49 Dermatomyositis, heliotrope. *Courtesy Ken Greer, MD.*

Fig. 8.50 Dermatomyositis, heliotrope.

Fig. 8.51 Dermatomyositis, Gottron's papules.

Fig. 8.52 Dermatomyositis, Gottron's papules.

Fig. 8.53 Dermatomyositis, Gottron's papules.

Fig. 8.54 Dermatomyositis, frayed cuticles (Samitz sign).

Fig. 8.55 Dermatomyositis, Gottron's sign.

Fig. 8.56 Dermatomyositis, Gottron's sign.

Fig. 8.57 Dermatomyositis, shawl sign. *Courtesy Steven Binnick, MD.*

Fig. 8.58 Dermatomyositis, shawl sign.

Fig. 8.59 Dermatomyositis, shawl sign.

Fig. 8.60 Dermatomyositis.

Fig. 8.61 Dermatomyositis.

Fig. 8.62 Dermatomyositis, mechanic's hands.

Fig. 8.63 Dermatomyositis with calcification. *Courtesy Steven Binnick, MD.*

Fig. 8.64 Dermatomyositis with ulceration.

Fig. 8.65 Morphea.

Fig. 8.66 Morphea.

Fig. 8.67 Morphea with lichen sclerosis overlap.

Fig. 8.68 Generalized morphea.

Fig. 8.69 Atrophoderma of Pasini and Pierini.

Fig. 8.70 Atrophoderma of Pasini and Pierini.

Fig. 8.71 Linear morphea. *Courtesy Debabrata Bandyopadhyay, MD.*

Fig. 8.72 Linear morphea. *Courtesy Lisa Arkin, MD.*

Fig. 8.73 Linear morphea.

Fig. 8.74 Parry-Romberg syndrome.

Fig. 8.75 Sclerodactyly in limited scleroderma, CREST.

Fig. 8.76 Sclerodactyly and Delangiectasias in limited scleroderma, CREST.

Fig. 8.77 Calcinosis of the knee in a patient with scleroderma.

Fig. 8.78 Sclerodactyly in systemic sclerosis.

Fig. 8.79 Sclerotic digit (L) versus normal digit (R).

Fig. 8.80 Sclerodactyly with ulcerations in systemic sclerosis.

Fig. 8.81 Ulceration in systemic sclerosis.

Fig. 8.82 Telangiectasias in systemic sclerosis.

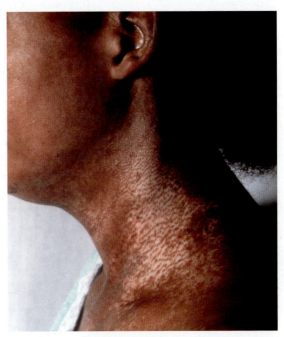

Fig. 8.83 Dyspigmentation in systemic sclerosis.

Fig. 8.84 Eosinophilic fasciitis.

Fig. 8.85 Eosinophilic fasciitis.

Fig. 8.86 Mixed connective tissue disease. *Courtesy Steven Binnick, MD.*

Fig. 8.87 Mixed connective tissue disease. *Courtesy Steven Binnick, MD.*

Fig. 8.88 Nephrogenic systemic fibrosis.

Fig. 8.89 Nephrogenic systemic fibrosis.

Fig. 8.90 Sjogren syndrome.

Fig. 8.91 Annular erythema of Sjogren syndrome.

Fig. 8.92 Rheumatoid nodules.

Fig. 8.93 Rheumatoid nodules.

Fig. 8.94 Rheumatoid vasculitis.

Fig. 8.95 Rheumatoid vasculitis.

Fig. 8.96 Still's disease.

Fig. 8.97 Relapsing polychondritis.

Fig. 8.98 Relapsing polychondritis.

Mucinoses 9

Localized cutaneous mucin deposition results in translucent pale to erythematous papules, as in digital myxoid cysts or focal cutaneous mucinosis. Papular mucinosis related to plasma cell dyscrasia with paraproteinemia causes papules with a distinct tendency to form linear arrays. Histologically, mucin is less apparent than an increase in fibroblasts and ropey collagen. This translates to induration of the skin over time, leading to a clinical appearance resembling systemic sclerosis.

Myxedema results in subtle dermal mucin deposition often manifesting below the eyes, whereas pretibial myxedema can produce dramatic deposition within the skin of the dorsal foot as well as the pretibial region. Stasis-induced mucinosis can produce a similar appearance, but the mucin is confined to the upper dermis rather than affecting the full thickness of the dermis as is seen in thyroid disease.

Follicular mucinosis can occur as erythematous, indurated, hairless plaques in benign alopecia mucinosa, as well as in the setting of mycosis fungoides. Dilated follicular orifices can give the appearance of comedones (blackheads), and sticky gelatinous material may be extruded from the lesions. This portion of the atlas will guide you through the various clinical presentations associated with mucinosis.

Fig. 9.1 Early scleromyxedema.

Fig. 9.2 Scleromyxedema.

Fig. 9.3 Scleromyxedema. *Courtesy Robert Lee, MD.*

Fig. 9.4 Scleromyxedema.

Fig. 9.5 (A) Scleromyxedema. *Courtesy Douglas Pugliese, MD.*
(B) Scleromyxedema. *Courtesy Douglas Pugliese, MD.*

Fig. 9.6 Scleromyxedema. *Courtesy Douglas Pugliese, MD.*

Fig. 9.7 Scleromyxedema. *Courtesy Rui Tavares Bello, MD.*

Fig. 9.8 Scleromyxedema. *Courtesy Douglas Pugliese, MD.*

Fig. 9.9 (A) Acral persistent papular mucinosis. *Courtesy Juliana Choi, MD and Iris K. Aronson, MD.* (B) Acral persistent papular mucinosis. *Courtesy Juliana Choi, MD and Iris K. Aronson, MD.*

Fig. 9.10 Mucinous papules in an HIV-positive patient.

Fig. 9.11 Self-healing papular mucinosis.

Fig. 9.12 Scleredema. *Courtesy Steven Binnick, MD.*

Fig. 9.13 Scleredema.

Fig. 9.14 Reticular erythematous mucinosis.

Fig. 9.15 Reticular erythematous mucinosis.

Fig. 9.16 Benign follicular mucinosis. *Courtesy Rui Tavares Bello, MD.*

Fig. 9.17 Benign follicular mucinosis. *Courtesy Steven Binnick, MD.*

Fig. 9.18 Benign follicular mucinosis. *Courtesy Steven Binnick, MD.*

Fig. 9.19 Benign follicular mucinosis. *Courtesy Scott Norton, MD.*

Fig. 9.20 Benign follicular mucinosis. *Courtesy Steven Binnick, MD.*

Fig. 9.21 Follicular mucinosis associated with mycosis fungoides.

Fig. 9.22 Follicular mucinosis associated with mycosis fungoides.

Fig. 9.23 Follicular mucinosis associated with mycosis fungoides. *Courtesy Ellen Kim, MD.*

Fig. 9.24 Focal cutaneous mucinosis.

Fig. 9.25 Myxoid cyst. *Courtesy Steven Binnick, MD.*

Fig. 9.26 Myxoid cyst. Note nail deformity. *Courtesy Steven Binnick, MD.*

Seborrheic Dermatitis, Psoriasis, Recalcitrant Palmoplantar Eruptions, Pustular Dermatitis, and Erythroderma

10

The primary lesion of a papulosquamous disorder is a papule with scale, but because patients often present later in the course of disease, the primary lesions may not be visible, and the physician may observe scaly plaques, patches, postinflammatory change, or diffuse redness and scaling (erythroderma).

Seborrheic dermatitis may involve the eyebrows, nasolabial and melolabial folds, scalp, ears, retroauricular regions, central chest, and axillae. The scale often exhibits a yellow hue, most likely related to carotenoids within the serum crusts. This is in stark contrast to the silvery white scale of typical plaque psoriasis. Plaque psoriasis lacks spongiosis (and the yellow carotenoids that are dissolved in the aqueous phase of tissue fluids). Several forms of psoriasis exhibit spongiosis and can sometimes have a slightly yellow appearance to the scale. These include guttate, inverse, acral, and erythrodermic forms of psoriasis. Even in these forms, frankly yellow scale and honey crusts are rare.

Erythroderma presents with generalized erythema and scaling. Edema may be present, especially involving the face and extremities, and patients may suffer chills as a result of loss of body heat. Older patients may exhibit signs of high-output cardiac failure. This portion of the atlas will guide you through the various clinical manifestations of seborrheic dermatitis, psoriasis, and related disorders.

Fig. 10.1 Seborrheic dermatitis.

Fig. 10.2 Seborrheic dermatitis.

Fig. 10.3 Seborrheic dermatitis.

Fig. 10.4 Seborrheic dermatitis. *Courtesy Steven Binnick, MD.*

Fig. 10.5 Seborrheic dermatitis. *Courtesy Steven Binnick, MD.*

Fig. 10.6 Seborrheic dermatitis in an HIV-positive patient.

Fig. 10.7 Cradle cap.

Fig. 10.8 Seborrheic dermatitis with hyperpigmentation in an African American patient.

Fig. 10.9 Seborrheic dermatitis with hypopigmentation in an African American patient. *Courtesy Scott Norton, MD.*

Fig. 10.10 Psoriasis.

Fig. 10.11 Psoriasis.

Fig. 10.12 Psoriasis.

Fig. 10.13 Psoriasis.

Fig. 10.14 Psoriasis.

Fig. 10.15 Psoriasis.

Fig. 10.16 Psoriasis.

Fig. 10.17 Psoriasis.

Fig. 10.18 Psoriasis.

Fig. 10.19 Psoriasis.

Fig. 10.20 Psoriasis.

Fig. 10.21 Psoriasis.

Fig. 10.22 Psoriasis.

Fig. 10.23 Psoriasis.

Fig. 10.24 Psoriasis. *Courtesy Shyam Verma, MBBS, DVD.*

Fig. 10.25 Psoriasis. *Courtesy Steven Binnick, MD.*

Fig. 10.26 Psoriasis.

Fig. 10.27 Psoriasis.

Fig. 10.28 Psoriasis. *Courtesy Steven Binnick, MD.*

Fig. 10.29 Psoriasis. *Courtesy Steven Binnick, MD.*

Fig. 10.30 Psoriasis.

Fig. 10.31 Psoriasis.

Fig. 10.32 Nail pitting in psoriasis.

Fig. 10.33 Oil spot and subungual hyperkeratosis in nail psoriasis.

Fig. 10.34 Nail psoriasis.

Fig. 10.35 Nail psoriasis.

Fig. 10.36 Inverse psoriasis.

Fig. 10.37 Inverse psoriasis. *Courtesy Steven Binnick, MD.*

Fig. 10.38 Infantile psoriasis.

Fig. 10.39 Infantile psoriasis. *Courtesy Paul Honig, MD.*

Fig. 10.40 Infantile psoriasis.

Fig. 10.41 Guttate psoriasis.

Fig. 10.42 Guttate psoriasis.

Fig. 10.43 Guttate psoriasis.

Fig. 10.44 Linear psoriasis.

Fig. 10.45 Psoriasis after zoster in an HIV-infected patient. *Courtesy Vikash Oza, MD.*

Fig. 10.46 Annular psoriasis.

Fig. 10.47 Pustular psoriasis.

Fig. 10.48 Pustular psoriasis.

Fig. 10.49 Pustular psoriasis.

Fig. 10.50 Pustular psoriasis.

Fig. 10.51 Erythrodermic psoriasis.

Fig. 10.52 Erythrodermic psoriasis.

Fig. 10.53 Hands in erythrodermic psoriasis.

Fig. 10.54 Psoriatic arthritis. *Courtesy Steven Binnick, MD.*

Fig. 10.55 Psoriatic arthritis.

Fig. 10.56 Reactive arthritis with oral erythema.

Fig. 10.57 Reactive arthritis with urethral inflammation.

Fig. 10.59 Reactive arthritis.

Fig. 10.58 Reactive arthritis with conjunctival erythema.

Fig. 10.60 Reactive arthritis.

Fig. 10.61 Reactive arthritis.

Fig. 10.62 Reactive arthritis.

Fig. 10.63 Reactive arthritis.

Fig. 10.64 Reactive arthritis.

Fig. 10.65 Subcorneal pustular dermatosis.

Fig. 10.66 Subcorneal pustular dermatosis.

Fig. 10.67 Subcorneal pustular dermatosis. *Courtesy Steven Binnick, MD.*

Fig. 10.68 Papuloerythroderma of Ofuji. *Courtesy of Department of Dermatology, Keio University School of Medicine, Tokyo, Japan.*

Fig. 10.69 Pediatric eosinophilic pustular folliculitis. *Courtesy Paul Honig, MD.*

Fig. 10.70 Pediatric eosinophilic pustular folliculitis.

Fig. 10.71 Acrodermatitis continua.

Fig. 10.72 Acrodermatitis continua.

Fig. 10.73 Acrodermatitis continua. *Courtesy Steven Binnick, MD.*

Fig. 10.74 Recurrent palmoplantar pustulosis.

Fig. 10.75 Palmoplantar pustulosis.

Fig. 10.76 Palmoplantar pustulosis. *Courtesy Steven Binnick, MD.*

Fig. 10.77 Palmoplantar pustulosis.

Fig. 10.78 Palmoplantar pustulosis.

Fig. 10.79 Acropustulosis of infancy.

Pityriasis Rosea, Pityriasis Rubra Pilaris, and Other Papulosquamous and Hyperkeratotic Diseases

Pityriasis rosea presents with erythematous macules that develop a delicate central silver scale. As the lesions evolve, they assume an oval configuration often best observed on the back and flanks. The scale becomes a peripheral collarette as the lesions evolve. Histologically, erythrocyte extravasation is characteristic, and clinically purpuric lesions may occasionally be noted. In patients with darker skin, the lesions of pityriasis rosea may assume a papular appearance. A more characteristic oval character is often evident on the upper flank near the axillary vault and can be helpful in confirming the diagnosis.

Pityriasis rubra pilaris (PRP) may present with classic nutmeg-grater, spiky, keratotic papules involving the dorsal digits, or may present with more subtle erythema and scale involving the hands, face, and scalp. Evolution can be rapid, and the patient can assume the appearance of erythroderma with characteristic islands of sparing. The eruptions often have a distinctly orange appearance, especially on the palms. Juvenile forms of PRP can present with nummular arrays of spiky papules or with hyperkeratotic plaques involving the extensors in a pattern reminiscent of psoriasis. Discrete keratotic follicular papules are often present at the periphery and are helpful in establishing the correct diagnosis without the need for biopsy. This portion of the atlas will guide you through the various clinical presentations of these disorders.

Fig. 11.1 Small plaque parapsoriasis.

Fig. 11.2 Digitate parapsoriasis.

Fig. 11.3 Confluent and reticulated papillomatosis.

Fig. 11.4 Confluent and reticulated papillomatosis.

Fig. 11.5 Confluent and reticulated papillomatosis. *Courtesy Steven Binnick, MD.*

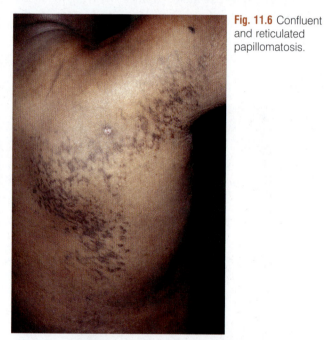

Fig. 11.6 Confluent and reticulated papillomatosis.

Fig. 11.7 Confluent and reticulated papillomatosis.

Fig. 11.8 Confluent and reticulated papillomatosis.

Fig. 11.9 Pityriasis rosea herald patch. *Courtesy Steven Binnick, MD.*

Fig. 11.10 Pityriasis rosea herald patch.

Fig. 11.11 Pityriasis rosea.

Fig. 11.12 Pityriasis rosea. *Courtesy Steven Binnick, MD.*

Fig. 11.13 Pityriasis rosea.

Fig. 11.14 Pityriasis rosea.

Fig. 11.15 Pityriasis rubra pilaris with early follicular hyperkeratosis.

Fig. 11.16 Pityriasis rubra pilaris. *Courtesy Steven Binnick, MD.*

Fig. 11.17 Pityriasis rubra pilaris.

Fig. 11.18 Pityriasis rubra pilaris.

Fig. 11.19 Pityriasis rubra pilaris. *Courtesy Steven Binnick, MD.*

Fig. 11.20 Pityriasis rubra pilaris.

Fig. 11.21 Pityriasis rubra pilaris. *Courtesy Steven Binnick, MD.*

Fig. 11.22 Pityriasis rubra pilaris.

Fig. 11.23 Pityriasis rubra pilaris.

Fig. 11.24 Pityriasis rubra pilaris.

Fig. 11.25 Pityriasis rubra pilaris.

Fig. 11.26 Pityriasis rubra pilaris. *Courtesy Steven Binnick, MD.*

Fig. 11.27 Pityriasis rubra pilaris.

Fig. 11.28 Pityriasis rubra pilaris. *Courtesy Steven Binnick, MD.*

Fig. 11.29 Pityriasis rubra pilaris.

Fig. 11.30 Childhood pityriasis rubra pilaris.

Fig. 11.31 Childhood pityriasis rubra pilaris.

Fig. 11.32 Childhood pityriasis rubra pilaris.

Fig. 11.33 Circumscribed juvenile pityriasis rubra pilaris.

Fig. 11.34 Circumscribed juvenile pityriasis rubra pilaris.

Fig. 11.35 Circumscribed juvenile pityriasis rubra pilaris.

Fig. 11.36 Keratolysis exfoliativa.

Fig. 11.37 Keratolysis exfoliativa.

Fig. 11.38 Keratosis punctata of the palmar creases.

Fig. 11.39 Keratosis punctata of the palmar creases.

Fig. 11.40 Punctate keratoderma.

Fig. 11.41 Punctate keratoderma.

Fig. 11.42 Punctate keratoderma.

Fig. 11.43 Spiny hyperkeratosis of the palms.

Fig. 11.44 Keratoderma climactericum.

Fig. 11.45 Ichthyosis hystrix of Curth-Macklin with keratin 1 mutation.

Fig. 11.46 Diffuse hyperkeratosis of the palms, Unna-Thost.

Fig. 11.47 Diffuse hyperkeratosis of the palms, Unna-Thost.

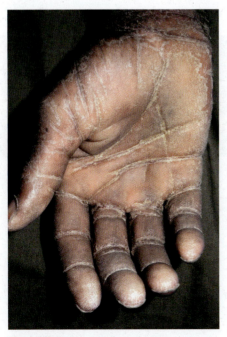

Fig. 11.48 Tylosis with lung cancer.

Fig. 11.49 Mutilating keratoderma of Vohwinkel.

Fig. 11.50 Mutilating keratoderma of Vohwinkel.

Fig. 11.51 Olmsted syndrome. *Courtesy Debabrata Bandyopadhyay.*

Fig. 11.52 Acrokeratoelastoidosis.

Fig. 11.53 Acrokeratoelastoidosis.

Fig. 11.54 Collagenous and elastotic marginal plaques of the hands.

Fig. 11.55 Focal acral hyperkeratosis.

Fig. 11.56 Focal acral hyperkeratosis.

Fig. 11.57 Mal de Meleda. *Courtesy Curt Samlaska, MD.*

Fig. 11.58 Mal de Meleda. *Courtesy Curt Samlaska, MD.*

Fig. 11.59 Papillon-Lefevre syndrome. *Courtesy Ken Greer, MD.*

Fig. 11.60 Papillon-Lefevre syndrome. *Courtesy Ken Greer, MD.*

Fig. 11.61 Papillon-Lefevre syndrome. *Courtesy Ken Greer, MD.*

Fig. 11.62 Papillon-Lefevre syndrome. *Courtesy Ken Greer, MD.*

Fig. 11.63 Striate keratoderma.

Fig. 11.64 Aquagenic wrinkling after immersing patient's left hand in water. First published in Katz KA, Yan AC, Turner ML: Aquagenic wrinkling of the palms in patients with cystic fibrosis homozygous for the delta F508 CFTR mutation. Arch Dermatol 2005: 141: 621-4.

Fig. 11.65 Aquagenic wrinkling after immersing the patient's left hand in water. First published in Katz KA, Yan AC, Turner ML: Aquagenic wrinkling of the palms in patients with cystic fibrosis homozygous for the delta F508 CFTR mutation. Arch Dermatol 2005: 141: 621-4.

Fig. 11.66 Erythroderma from atopic dermatitis.

Fig. 11.67 Psoriatic erythroderma.

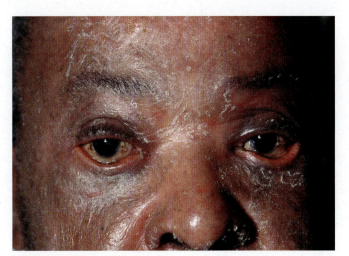

Fig. 11.68 Psoriatic erythroderma.

Lichen Planus and Related Conditions   12

Lichen planus (LP) and other lichenoid eruptions tend to create characteristic primary lesions and patterns. The pruritic, purple, polygonal, flat-topped papules of LP can appear unmistakably shiny as they reflect light back at the keen diagnostician. These papules can be widespread and coalesce into plaques and streaks that demonstrate the Koebner phenomenon as another clue to the diagnosis. A thorough physical examination can reveal white lacy leukoplakia of the oral mucosa, annular lesions of the genitalia, or a variety of nail changes from ridging to pterygium formation. Lichen planus pigmentosus/actinicus is an often photodistributed LP variant that demonstrates more distinctive hyperpigmentation.

Lichen nitidus and lichen striatus are lichenoid conditions that are more common in children. With its almost pinpoint, shiny, flat-topped papules, lichen nitidus can appear slightly hypopigmented against darker skin. As in LP, papules can demonstrate the Koebner phenomenon and be either localized or widespread. Lichen striatus presents with a characteristically curvilinear plaque most commonly on the extremities of a child; however, lesions can be seen on the trunk and, rarely, the face. The eruption follows the lines of Blaschko and can involve the nail with longitudinal dystrophy. In the later phase, a hypopigmented or hyperpigmented patch will remain on the skin temporarily as a sign of the recently resolved plaque of lichen striatus.

Lichen sclerosus most commonly involves the genitalia, with a higher incidence in females. Genital lichen sclerosus classically presents with atrophic white patches that can appear wrinkled and erosive, and can obliterate and scar normal anatomic landmarks. In some patients, the presence of bruising can be misdiagnosed as trauma from sexual abuse, highlighting the importance of a careful physical examination with consideration of skin biopsy in unclear cases. Extragenital lichen sclerosus can present with atrophic white papules and macules, often on the trunk.

Skin biopsy can be diagnostic in many lichenoid conditions, demonstrating the typical bandlike inflammation at the dermal-epidermal junction, along with more specific differentiating features depending on the specific eruption. This portion of the atlas features many images to help clinically distinguish lichen planus and its many related conditions.

Fig. 12.1 Lichen planus. *Courtesy Steven Binnick, MD.*

Fig. 12.2 Lichen planus.

Fig. 12.3 Lichen planus.

Fig. 12.4 Lichen planus.

Fig. 12.5 Lichen planus. *Courtesy Steven Binnick, MD.*

Fig. 12.6 Lichen planus.

Fig. 12.7 Lichen planus.

Fig. 12.8 Lichen planus.

Fig. 12.9 Lichen planus. *Courtesy Steven Binnick, MD.*

Fig. 12.10 Lichen planus. Note Koebner phenomenon.

Fig. 12.11 Lichen planus. *Courtesy Steven Binnick, MD.*

Fig. 12.12 Lichen planus. *Courtesy Ken Greer, MD.*

Fig. 12.13 Lichen planus.

Fig. 12.14 Lichen planus.

Fig. 12.15 Lichen planus.

Fig. 12.17 Lichen planus.

Fig. 12.16 Lichen planus. *Courtesy Steven Binnick, MD.*

Fig. 12.18 Hypertrophic lichen planus.

Fig. 12.19 Hypertrophic lichen planus.

Fig. 12.20 Hypertrophic lichen planus. *Courtesy Debabrata Bandyopadhyay, MD.*

Fig. 12.21 Lichen planus, glans penis.

Fig. 12.23 Lichen planus.

Fig. 12.22 Lichen planus.

Fig. 12.24 Lichen planus.

Fig. 12.25 Vulvovaginal-gingival syndrome.

Fig. 12.26 Vulvovaginal-gingival syndrome.

Fig. 12.27 Oral lichen planus.

Fig. 12.28 Oral lichen planus.

Fig. 12.29 Oral lichen planus.

Fig. 12.30 Oral lichen planus.

Fig. 12.31 Lip lichen planus. *Courtesy Steven Binnick, MD.*

Fig. 12.32 Erosive lichen planus. *Courtesy Steven Binnick, MD.*

Fig. 12.33 Lichen planus.

Fig. 12.34 Lichen planus.

Fig. 12.35 Lichen planus of the nail.

Fig. 12.36 Lichen planus of the nail.

Lichen planus and related conditions

Fig. 12.37 Lichen planus of the nails.

Fig. 12.38 Annular lichen planus. *Courtesy Steven Binnick, MD.*

Fig. 12.39 Annular lichen planus.

Fig. 12.40 Annular lichen planus.

Fig. 12.41 Annular lichen planus.

Fig. 12.42 Atrophic lichen planus.

Fig. 12.43 Eyelid lichen planus.

Fig. 12.44 Lichen planus after radiation therapy.

Fig. 12.45 Lichen planopilaris.

Fig. 12.46 Lichen planopilaris.

Fig. 12.47 Lichen planopilaris.

Fig. 12.48 Frontal fibrosing alopecia. *Courtesy Len Sperling, MD.*

Fig. 12.49 Graham-Little-Piccardi syndrome nonscarring hair loss of the trunk.

Fig. 12.50 Graham-Little-Piccardi syndrome nonscarring hair loss of the trunk.

Fig. 12.51 Lichen planus pigmentosa.

Fig. 12.52 Lichen planus actinicus. *Courtesy Steven Binnick, MD.*

Fig. 12.53 Lichen planus actinicus.

Fig. 12.54 Erythema dyschromicum persitans.

Fig. 12.55 Erythema dyschromicum perstans.

Fig. 12.56 Idiopathic eruptive macular hyperpigmentation with papillomatosis. *Courtesy Dr. Ang Chia Chun.*

Fig. 12.57 Idiopathic eruptive macular hyperpigmentation with papillomatosis. *Courtesy Dr. Ang Chia Chun.*

Fig. 12.58 Lichen nitidus.

Fig. 12.59 Lichen nitidus.

Fig. 12.60 Lichen nitidus.

Fig. 12.61 Lichen nitidus.

Fig. 12.62 Lichen nitidus. *Courtesy Curt Samlaska, MD.*

Fig. 12.63 Lichen nitidus. *Courtesy Curt Samlaska, MD.*

Fig. 12.64 Lichen nitidus.

Fig. 12.65 Lichen nitidus.

Fig. 12.66 Lichen nitidus.

Fig. 12.67 Lichen nitidus. *Courtesy Omar Noor, MD.*

Fig. 12.68 Lichen nitidus.

Fig. 12.69 Lichen nitidus. Note Koebner phenomenon. *Courtesy Curt Samlaska, MD.*

Fig. 12.70 Lichen striatus.

Fig. 12.71 Lichen striatus.

Fig. 12.72 Lichen striatus. *Courtesy Curt Samlaska, MD.*

Fig. 12.73 Lichen striatus.

Fig. 12.74 Lichen striatus.

Fig. 12.75 Lichen striatus.

Fig. 12.76 Lichen sclerosus et atrophicus.

Fig. 12.77 Lichen sclerosus et atrophicus. *Courtesy Ken Greer, MD.*

Fig. 12.78 Lichen sclerosus et atrophicus. *Courtesy Steven Binnick, MD.*

Fig. 12.79 Lichen sclerosus et atrophicus. *Courtesy Ken Greer, MD.*

Fig. 12.80 Lichen sclerosus et atrophicus, with hemorrhage secondary to atrophy and trauma.

Fig. 12.81 Lichen sclerosus et atrophicus.

Fig. 12.82 Lichen sclerosus et atrophicus. *Courtesy Shyam Verma, MBBS, DVD.*

Fig. 12.83 Lichen sclerosus et atrophicus.

Fig. 12.84 Lichen sclerosus et atrophicus.

Fig. 12.85 Lichen sclerosus et atrophicus.

Fig. 12.86 Lichen sclerosus et atrophicus, with hemorrhage secondary to atrophy and trauma.

Fig. 12.87 Lichen sclerosus et atrophicus. *Note Koebner phenomena.*

Fig. 12.88 Lichen sclerosus et atrophicus.

Acne 13

Typical acne is so commonplace that its comedones, papules, and pustules are immediately recognizable. There exist, however, a wide spectrum of acne lesions, acneiform eruptions, and rosacea that are exhibited here to assist the deciphering medical provider.

The earliest lesions of acne are open and closed comedones that are often first present on the forehead of adolescent patients. Papules, pustules, nodules, cysts, and scarring can also be seen in the typical acne-prone anatomic regions of the face, upper back, chest, shoulders, and upper arms. The most severe form of acne, acne fulminans, is characterized by joint pains, painful nodulocystic lesions, and even fevers. Other acneiform eruptions include the scarring follicular pustules of acne keloidalis nuchae, the more monomorphous pustular eruption of corticosteroid-induced acne, and the pustules and nodules of gram-negative folliculitis.

In neonates, the transient micropustular eruption on the head and neck that has been historically known as *neonatal acne* has now been renamed *neonatal cephalic pustulosis* due to its lack of comedones, nodules, or scarring. Infantile acne, in contrast, occurs mostly on the cheeks of infants and toddlers and is a true subset of acne with its comedones, papules, pustules, nodules, and potential scarring. Finally, periorificial dermatitis is a distinctive acneiform eruption notable for papules and pustules located around the mouth, nose, and eyes of children and younger adults.

Hidradenitis suppurativa is also included in this chapter with its chronic inflammatory abscesses, nodules, and sinus tract formation in the axillae, inframammary folds, inguinal folds, and gluteal cleft.

Rosacea is also highlighted here to allow for direct comparison with acne. Flushing, erythema, and fine telangiectasias seen on the convex surfaces of the face define the erythrotelangiectatic subtype of rosacea, whereas the papules, pustules, and in some cases nodules are present in the papulopustular and glandular forms.

Most conditions in this chapter will depend on clinical findings to arrive at a diagnosis, but in some cases a skin biopsy or bacterial culture will be useful. This portion of the atlas features examples of important clinical findings to recognize in patients with acne and the many acneiform eruptions.

Fig. 13.2 Neonatal cephalic pustulosis (neonatal acne).

Fig. 13.1 Neonatal cephalic pustulosis (neonatal acne).

Fig. 13.3 Neonatal cephalic pustulosis (neonatal acne).

Fig. 13.4 Infantile acne.

Fig. 13.5 Infantile acne.

Fig. 13.6 Severe infantile acne.

Fig. 13.7 Childhood acne.

Fig. 13.8 Childhood acne.

Fig. 13.9 Open comedones. *Courtesy Steven Binnick, MD.*

Fig. 13.20 Acne cyst with scarring. *Courtesy Steven Binnick, MD.*

Fig. 13.21 Severe acne.

Fig. 13.22 Severe truncal acne. *Courtesy Steven Binnick, MD.*

Fig. 13.23 Severe truncal acne.

Fig. 13.24 Severe truncal acne with hyperpigmentation.

Fig. 13.25 Acne with hyperpigmentation.

Fig. 13.26 Adult woman with lower face acne.

Fig. 13.27 Adult woman with lower face acne.

Fig. 13.28 Adult woman with lower face acne.

Fig. 13.29 Acne in woman with 21-hydroxylase deficiency. *Courtesy Steven Binnick, MD.*

Fig. 13.30 Acne and hirsutism in a woman with Cushing disease.

Fig. 13.31 Acne fulminans.

Fig. 13.10 Open comedones.

Fig. 13.11 Closed comedones.

Fig. 13.12 Closed comedones.

Fig. 13.13 Preadolescent acne.

Fig. 13.14 Preadolescent acne.

Fig. 13.15 Mild to moderate acne.

Fig. 13.16 Mild to moderate acne.

Fig. 13.17 Moderate to severe acne.

Fig. 13.18 Severe acne.

Fig. 13.19 Severe acne.

Fig. 13.32 Acne fulminans.

Fig. 13.33 Acne scarring. *Courtesy Steven Binnick, MD.*

Fig. 13.34 Acne scarring. *Courtesy Steven Binnick, MD.*

Fig. 13.35 Keloids resulting from acne. *Courtesy Steven Binnick, MD.*

Fig. 13.36 Solid facial edema.

Fig. 13.37 Osteoma cutis.

Fig. 13.38 Granulation tissue in a patient on isotretinoin. *Courtesy Steven Binnick, MD.*

Fig. 13.39 Minocycline pigmentation in an acne patient.

Fig. 13.40 Acne excoriée.

Fig. 13.41 Acne mechanica.

Fig. 13.42 Pomade acne.

Fig. 13.43 Acne cosmetica.

Fig. 13.44 Steroid acne in patient on oral steroids after neurosurgery.

Fig. 13.46 Steroid acne.

Fig. 13.48 Gram-negative folliculitis.

Fig. 13.45 Steroid acne.

Fig. 13.47 Chloracne.

Fig. 13.49 Gram-negative folliculitis.

Fig. 13.50 Gram-negative folliculitis.

Fig. 13.51 Acne keloidalis. *Courtesy Steven Binnick, MD.*

Fig. 13.52 Acne keloidalis.

Fig. 13.53 Hidradenitis suppurativa.

Fig. 13.54 Hidradenitis suppurativa.

Fig. 13.56 Hidradenitis suppurativa.

Fig. 13.55 Hidradenitis suppurativa. *Courtesy Steven Binnick, MD.*

Fig. 13.57 Hidradenitis suppurativa.

Fig. 13.58 Hidradenitis suppurativa.

Fig. 13.59 Hidradenitis suppurativa. *Courtesy Steven Binnick, MD.*

Fig. 13.60 Dissecting cellulitis of the scalp.

Fig. 13.61 Dissecting cellulitis of the scalp.

Fig. 13.62 Erythematotelangiectatic rosacea.

Fig. 13.63 Erythematotelangiectatic rosacea.

Fig. 13.64 Papulopustular rosacea.

Fig. 13.65 Papulopustular rosacea.

Fig. 13.66 Glandular rosacea.

Fig. 13.67 Glandular rosacea.

Fig. 13.68 Glandular rosacea with rhinophyma.

Fig. 13.69 Glandular rosacea with rhinophyma.

Fig. 13.70 Edema from rosacea (Morbihan disease).

Fig. 13.71 Pyoderma faciale.

Fig. 13.72 Pyoderma faciale. *Courtesy Steven Binnick, MD.*

Fig. 13.73 Perioral dermatitis.

Fig. 13.74 Perioral dermatitis. *Courtesy Steven Binnick, MD.*

Fig. 13.75 Rosacea induced by topical steroids.

Fig. 13.76 Granulomatous facial dermatitis.

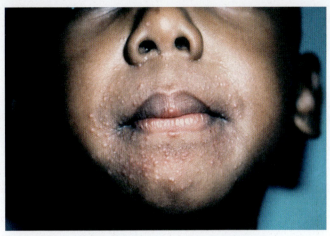

Fig. 13.78 Granulomatous facial dermatitis. *Courtesy Ken Greer, MD.*

Fig. 13.77 Granulomatous facial dermatitis.

Bacterial Infections 14

Bacterial infections create a multitude of skin lesions, from pustules, to necrotic nodules, to ulcers. These infections range from the superficial crusted erosions of impetigo to the systemic purpuric plaques of meningococcemia. This chapter categorizes these bacterial conditions into gram positive, gram negative, and others, including rickettsial diseases.

Recognizing the signs of bacterial infections is critical because most conditions will require treatment, whether topical or systemic. Staphylococcal skin infections can present with pustules, crusting, furuncles, or bullae in the case of bullous impetigo. Toxin-mediated conditions, such as staphylococcal scalded skin syndrome or toxic shock syndrome, will manifest as sunburn-like transient erythema accentuated in the folds. Streptococcal infections can present with pustules and crusting, as well as the firm painful erythematous plaques of cellulitis or erysipelas, or the ulcerative lesions in the case of ecthyma.

The anatomic locations involved can be a clue to which bacterial infections are most likely, such as in blistering distal dactylitis, perianal streptococcal infections, intertrigo, or gram-negative toe web infections.

Certain bacterial infections, along with deep fungal infections and atypical mycobacteria, should be included on the list of causes when evaluating a patient with isolated or multifocal necrotic dusky papules, nodules, ulcers, and eschars. This differential diagnosis is especially important in the setting of an immunocompromised host. These bacterial infections can include disseminated diseases from more common opportunistic organisms such as pseudomonas and those rarer conditions such as tularemia or anthrax.

Lastly, more distinctive conditions are included, such as the petechial exanthem of Rocky Mountain spotted fever, angiomatous papules of bacillary angiomatosis, and the expanding annular plaques of erythema migrans seen in Lyme disease.

Depending on the infections suspected, the workup for these conditions can include surface cultures, tissue cultures, and skin biopsy samples with subsequent special stains. This portion of the atlas contains images of common, uncommon, superficial, and disseminated bacterial infections and their many manifestations in the skin.

Fig. 14.1 Janeway spot in staphylococcal endocarditis. *Courtesy Curt Samlaska, MD.*

Fig. 14.2 Staphylococcal emboli from an infected iliac aneurysm. *Courtesy Curt Samlaska, MD.*

Fig. 14.3 Sycosis barbae. *Courtesy Steven Binnick, MD.*

Fig. 14.4 Staphylococcal folliculitis.

Fig. 14.5 Staphylococcal folliculitis.

Fig. 14.6 Staphylococcal folliculitis.

Fig. 14.7 Staphylococcal folliculitis.

Fig. 14.8 Staphylococcal folliculitis.

Fig. 14.9 Staphylococcal abscess. *Courtesy Steven Binnick, MD.*

Fig. 14.10 Staphylococcal abscess. *Courtesy Steven Binnick, MD.*

Fig. 14.11 Staphylococcal abscess.

Fig. 14.12 Subungual staphylococcal abscess. *Courtesy Ken Greer, MD.*

Fig. 14.13 Acute paronychia.

Fig. 14.14 Acute paronychia.

Fig. 14.15 Botryomycosis. *Courtesy Dermatology Division, University of Campinas, Brazil.*

Fig. 14.16 Botryomycosis. *Courtesy Tatiana C. P. Cordeiro de Andrade, MD.*

Fig. 14.17 Vegetating pyoderma.

Fig. 14.18 Vegetating pyoderma.

Fig. 14.19 Impetigo.

Fig. 14.20 Impetigo. *Courtesy Steven Binnick, MD.*

Fig. 14.21 Bullous impetigo.

Fig. 14.22 Bullous impetigo. *Courtesy Steven Binnick, MD.*

Fig. 14.23 Bullous impetigo. *Courtesy Steven Binnick, MD.*

Fig. 14.24 Early staphylococcal scalded skin syndrome. Note erythema accentuated in folds.

Fig. 14.25 Staphylococcal scalded skin syndrome.

Fig. 14.26 Staphylococcal scalded skin syndrome.

Fig. 14.27 Staphylococcal scalded skin syndrome.

Fig. 14.28 Ecthyma.

Fig. 14.29 Ecthyma. *Courtesy Curt Samlaska, MD.*

Fig. 14.30 Scarlet fever.

Fig. 14.31 Strawberry tongue.

Fig. 14.32 Erysipelas.

Fig. 14.33 Erysipelas.

Fig. 14.34 Erysipelas. *Courtesy Steven Binnick, MD.*

Fig. 14.35 Erysipelas.

Fig. 14.36 Cellulitis. *Courtesy Steven Binnick, MD.*

Fig. 14.37 Cellulitis. *Courtesy Steven Binnick, MD.*

Fig. 14.38 Early necrotizing fasciitis.

Fig. 14.39 Necrotizing fasciitis.

Fig. 14.40 Blistering dactylitis.

Fig. 14.41 Blistering dactylitis. *Courtesy Scott Norton, MD.*

Fig. 14.42 Perianal streptococcal infection.

Fig. 14.43 Streptococcal intertrigo. *Courtesy Paul Honig, MD.*

Fig. 14.44 Erythema marginatum. *Courtesy Steven Binnick, MD.*

Fig. 14.45 Erythema marginatum.

Fig. 14.46 Erysipeloid. *Courtesy Steven Binnick, MD.*

Fig. 14.47 Erysipeloid.

Fig. 14.48 Anthrax with severe edema. *Courtesy Steve Krivda, MD.*

Fig. 14.49 Cutaneous diphtheria.

Fig. 14.50 Erythrasma. *Courtesy Steven Binnick, MD.*

Fig. 14.51 Erythrasma.

Fig. 14.52 Intertrigo.

Fig. 14.53 Pitted keratolysis. *Courtesy Shyam Verma, MBBS, DVD.*

Fig. 14.54 Pitted keratolysis.

Fig. 14.55 Clostridial ulcer. *Courtesy Steven Binnick, MD.*

Fig. 14.56 Actinomycosis. *Courtesy Steven Binnick, MD.*

Fig. 14.57 Actinomycosis. *Courtesy Dermatology Division, University of Campinas, Brazil.*

Fig. 14.58 Nocardia.

Fig. 14.59 Nocardia. *Courtesy Curt Samlaska, MD.*

Fig. 14.60 Nocardia.

Fig. 14.61 Ecthyma gangrenosum.

Fig. 14.62 Ecthyma gangrenosum. *Courtesy Scott Norton, MD.*

Fig. 14.63 Green nail secondary to Pseudomonal infection. *Courtesy Steven Binnick, MD.*

Fig. 14.64 Gram-negative toe web infection.

Fig. 14.65 Gram-negative toe web infection. *Courtesy Ken Greer, MD.*

Fig. 14.66 Hot tub folliculitis. *Courtesy Steven Binnick, MD.*

Fig. 14.67 Hot tub folliculitis. *Courtesy Steven Binnick, MD.*

Fig. 14.68 Hot tub folliculitis. *Courtesy Steven Binnick, MD.*

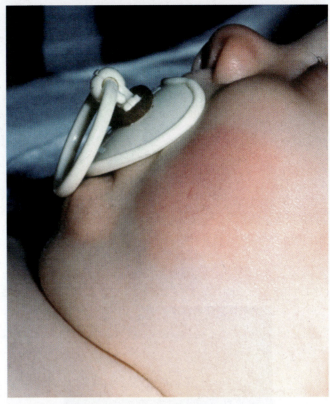

Fig. 14.69 *Haemophilus influenzae* cellulitis.

Fig. 14.70 Chancroid.

Fig. 14.71 Chancroid.

Fig. 14.72 Chancroid. *Courtesy Scott Norton, MD.*

Fig. 14.73 Granuloma inguinale.

Fig. 14.74 Granuloma inguinale.

Fig. 14.75 Gonococcal infection.

Fig. 14.76 Gonococcemia.

Fig. 14.77 Gonococcemia.

Fig. 14.78 Meningococcemia. *Courtesy Scott Norton, MD.*

Fig. 14.79 Meningococcemia.

Fig. 14.80 *Vibrio vulnificus* infection. *Courtesy Curt Samlaska, MD.*

Fig. 14.81 Rhinoscleroma. *Courtesy Steven Binnick, MD.*

Fig. 14.82 Infected human bite. *Courtesy Steven Binnick, MD.*

Fig. 14.83 Cat scratch disease.

Fig. 14.84 Bacillary angiomatosis.

Fig. 14.85 Bacillary angiomatosis.

Fig. 14.86 Verruga peruana. *Courtesy Steven Binnick, MD.*

Fig. 14.87 Tularemia. *Courtesy Ken Greer, MD.*

Fig. 14.88 Tularemia. *Courtesy Stephen D. Hess, MD, PhD.*

Fig. 14.89 Epidemic typhus. *Courtesy Richard DeVillez, MD.*

Fig. 14.90 Epidemic typhus. *Courtesy Richard DeVillez, MD.*

Fig. 14.91 Rocky Mountain spotted fever. *Courtesy Paul Honig, MD.*

Fig. 14.92 Boutonneuse fever.

Fig. 14.93 Tache noire.

Fig. 14.94 Rickettsial pox.

Fig. 14.95 Erythema migrans.

Fig. 14.96 Erythema migrans. *Courtesy Steven Binnick, MD.*

Fig. 14.97 Erythema migrans. *Courtesy Steven Binnick, MD.*

Fig. 14.98 Erythema migrans.

Fig. 14.99 Acrodermatitis chronica atrophicans. *Courtesy Jisun Cha, MD, Rutgers-Robert Wood Johnson Medical School.*

Fig. 14.100 Lymphogranuloma venereum.

Diseases Resulting From Fungi and Yeasts 15

Fungi and yeasts can cause both superficial and deep infections in the skin with a great variation in clinical findings. In healthy hosts, commensal organisms such as candida remain superficial, whereas in the setting of an immunocompromised host they can be opportunistic, disseminated, and in some, lethal. Being familiar with both the common and uncommon fungi and yeasts and how they can present in the skin is important to allow for early diagnosis and treatment.

Dermatophyte infections in the skin are common, often pruritic, and almost always demonstrate persistent erythema and scaling of the affected regions. Tinea capitis can present with alopecia, broken hairs, localized or diffuse, fine scalp scaling, pustules, or painful boggy plaques with reactive cervical or occipital lymphadenopathy. Tinea, like other fungi and yeasts, tends to involve moist anatomic locations such as the body folds (axillae and groin) and the nail folds. Tinea corporis and faciei classically display the telltale annular or arcuate expanding patches or thin plaques with prominent scale at the leading edges. Appreciating this annularity can be difficult in some anatomic sites that are more convex or complicated such as around the ears or nose. Similarly difficult is when topical corticosteroids are used inadvertently on cutaneous dermatophyte infections resulting in a misleading clinical appearance with less scaling and erythema.

Candidal infections in the skin are also diverse, resulting in oral leukoplakia (thrush); the fissuring and erythema of the oral commissures known as *angular cheilitis*; chronic paronychia; itching, erythema and white discharge of candidal vulvovaginitis; and the beefy red, erosive intertrigo of the folds with surrounding satellite pustules seen commonly in the diaper region of infants. In newborns, congenital candidiasis can take on multiple forms, including a widespread miliaria-like eruption, pustules, or erosions that are most likely self-limited in full-term patients, but can disseminate in those born prematurely.

Deep fungal and mold infections include those regional organisms that infect otherwise well patients, such as *Histoplasmosis* and *Coccidiomycosis*, and those opportunistic and ubiquitous pathogens such as *Fusarium*, *Aspergillosis*, and the zygomycoses. Although many of these fungi and molds can present with nonspecific skin lesions, including abscesses, ulcers, verrucous or hyperkeratotic plaques, or nodules with central crusts or eschars, some more specific eruptions are also seen with these infections. These more specific eruptions can be a clue to the underlying immune status of the patient, including erythema nodosum seen more commonly in immunocompetent patients with coccidiomycosis or histoplasmosis versus the disseminated molluscum-like papules seen more in immunocompromised patients with these same infections.

This portion of the atlas portrays the myriad of skin findings due to fungi and yeasts and how their appearance can vary depending on the underlying immune status of the host patient.

Fig. 15.1 Tinea capitis.

Fig. 15.2 Tinea capitis.

Fig. 15.3 Kerion. *Courtesy Steven Binnick, MD.*

Fig. 15.4 Kerion. *Courtesy Steven Binnick, MD.*

Fig. 15.5 Id reaction.

Fig. 15.6 Id reaction.

Fig. 15.7 Tinea barbae.

Fig. 15.8 Tinea barbae.

Fig. 15.9 Tinea faciei.

Fig. 15.10 Tinea faciei. *Courtesy Steven Binnick, MD.*

Fig. 15.11 Tinea corporis. *Courtesy Steven Binnick, MD.*

Fig. 15.12 Tinea corporis.

Fig. 15.13 Tinea corporis.

Fig. 15.14 Tinea corporis (due to M canis). *Courtesy Scott Norton, MD.*

Fig. 15.15 Majocchi granuloma.

Fig. 15.16 Majocchi granuloma.

Fig. 15.17 Majocchi granuloma.

Fig. 15.18 Tinea imbricata.

Fig. 15.19 Tinea cruris.

Fig. 15.20 Tinea cruris.

Fig. 15.21 Perianal tinea.

Fig. 15.22 Interdigital tinea.

Fig. 15.23 Tinea pedis. *Courtesy Steven Binnick, MD.*

Fig. 15.24 Tinea pedis. *Courtesy Steven Binnick, MD.*

Fig. 15.25 Tinea pedis.

Fig. 15.26 Bullous tinea pedis in a 22-month-old boy.

Fig. 15.27 Bullous tinea pedis.

Fig. 15.28 One hand involvement with tinea. Patient had both feet involved. *Courtesy Steven Binnick, MD.*

Fig. 15.29 Onychomycosis.

Fig. 15.30 Onychomycosis.

Fig. 15.31 Dermatophytoma.

Fig. 15.32 Thrush in chronic mucocutaneous candidiasis.

Fig. 15.33 Oral candidiasis in an HIV-infected patient.

Fig. 15.34 Perléche.

Fig. 15.35 Candidiasis. *Courtesy Steven Binnick, MD.*

Fig. 15.36 Candidiasis. *Courtesy Curt Samlaska, MD.*

Fig. 15.37 Candidiasis.

Fig. 15.38 Candidiasis. *Courtesy Curt Samlaska, MD.*

Fig. 15.39 Candidiasis. *Courtesy Curt Samlaska, MD.*

Fig. 15.40 Candidiasis.

Fig. 15.41 Candidiasis. *Courtesy Steven Binnick, MD.*

Fig. 15.42 Congenital candidiasis.

Fig. 15.43 Congenital candidiasis. *Courtesy Vikash Oza, MD.*

Fig. 15.44 Candidiasis. *Courtesy Curt Samlaska, MD.*

Fig. 15.45 Erosio interdigitalis blastomycetica.

Fig. 15.46 Chronic paronychia.

Fig. 15.47 Chronic mucocutaneous candidiasis.

Fig. 15.48 Chronic mucocutaneous candidiasis.

Fig. 15.49 Chronic mucocutaneous candidiasis.

Fig. 15.50 Candidal sepsis.

Fig. 15.51 Candidal sepsis.

Fig. 15.52 Candidal sepsis.

Fig. 15.53 Tinea nigra.

Fig. 15.54 Tinea versicolor.

Fig. 15.55 Tinea versicolor. *Courtesy Steven Binnick, MD.*

Fig. 15.56 Tinea versicolor. *Courtesy Steven Binnick, MD.*

Fig. 15.57 Tinea versicolor.

Fig. 15.58 Tinea versicolor. *Courtesy Steven Binnick, MD.*

Fig. 15.59 Tinea versicolor.

Fig. 15.60 Tinea versicolor.

Fig. 15.61 Tinea versicolor. *Courtesy Steven Binnick, MD.*

Fig. 15.62 Tinea versicolor. *Courtesy Steven Binnick, MD.*

Fig. 15.63 Pityrosporum folliculitis.

Fig. 15.64 Pityrosporum folliculitis.

Fig. 15.65 Coccidioidomycosis.

Fig. 15.66 Coccidioidomycosis.

Fig. 15.67 Coccidioidomycosis. *Courtesy Curt Samlaska, MD.*

Fig. 15.68 Histoplasmosis. *Courtesy Steven Binnick, MD.*

Fig. 15.69 Histoplasmosis. *Courtesy Shyam Verma, MBBS, DVD.*

Fig. 15.70 Histoplasmosis. *Courtesy Shyam Verma, MBBS, DVD.*

Diseases resulting from fungi and yeasts

Fig. 15.71 Cryptococcal infection in an HIV-infected patient. *Courtesy Michelle Weir, MD.*

Fig. 15.72 Cryptococcal infection.

Fig. 15.73 Cryptococcal infection.

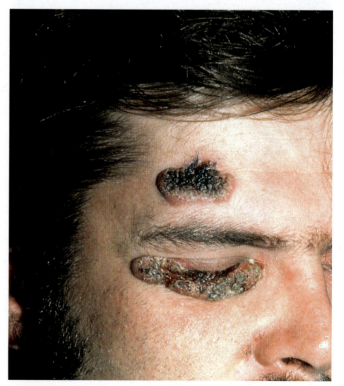

Fig. 15.74 North American blastomycosis.

Fig. 15.75 North American blastomycosis.

Fig. 15.76 Paracoccidiomycosis. *Courtesy Lauro de Souza Lima Institute, Brazil.*

Fig. 15.77 Paracoccidiomycosis. *Courtesy Lauro de Souza Lima Institute, Brazil.*

Fig. 15.78 Paracoccidiomycosis. *Courtesy Tatiana C. P. Cordeiro de Andrade, MD.*

Fig. 15.79 Paracoccidiomycosis. *Courtesy Lauro de Souza Lima Institute, Brazil.*

Fig. 15.80 Sporotrichosis. *Courtesy Lauro de Souza Lima Institute, Brazil.*

Fig. 15.81 Sporotrichosis. *Courtesy Lauro de Souza Lima Institute, Brazil.*

Fig. 15.82 Fixed cutaneous sporotrichosis. *Courtesy Scott Norton, MD.*

Fig. 15.83 Disseminated sporotrichosis. *Courtesy Scott Norton, MD.*

Fig. 15.84 Chromomycosis. *Courtesy Department of Dermatology, University of Campinas, Brazil.*

Fig. 15.86 Chromomycosis. *Courtesy Lauro de Souza Lima Institute, Brazil.*

Fig. 15.85 Chromomycosis. *Courtesy Lauro de Souza Lima Institute, Brazil.*

Fig. 15.87 Phaeohyphomycosis. *Courtesy Scott Norton, MD.*

Fig. 15.88 Phaeohyphomycosis.

Fig. 15.90 Mycetoma. *Courtesy Lauro de Souza Lima Institute, Brazil.*

Fig. 15.89 Mycetoma. *Courtesy Debabrata Bandyopadhyay, MD.*

Fig. 15.91 Mycetoma. *Courtesy Debabrata Bandyopadhyay, MD.*

Fig. 15.92 Lobomycosis. *Courtesy Lauro de Souza Lima Institute, Brazil.*

Fig. 15.93 Lobomycosis. *Courtesy Lauro de Souza Lima Institute, Brazil.*

Fig. 15.94 Mucormycosis.

Fig. 15.95 Zygomycosis at site of adhesive bandage.

Fig. 15.96 *Rhizopus* infection.

Fig. 15.97 *Fusarium* infection in a leukemic patient. Courtesy Curt Samlaska, MD.

Fig. 15.98 *Aspergillus* infection in a leukemic patient.

Fig. 15.99 *Aspergillus* infection in a leukemic patient.

Fig. 15.100 *Aspergillus* infection in a patient with chronic granulomatous disease.

Fig. 15.101 *Aspergillus* infection in a leukemic patient.

Mycobacterial Diseases 16

Tuberculosis and atypical mycobacterial infections can be difficult to diagnose clinically and require a high index of suspicion and familiarity with their manifestations in the skin.

Tuberculosis (TB) is more prevalent in the developing countries, especially those with particularly high rates of human immunodeficiency virus (HIV)–positive populations. The classification system of cutaneous TB depends on how the infection was acquired, and these four forms include many different cutaneous lesions. Examples of these four categories include 1) verrucous papules or plaques of primary inoculation TB (TB verrucosa cutis); 2) masses and nodules with possible suppuration and ulceration overlying infected lymph nodes representing endogenous, contiguous spread; 3) widespread macules, papules, pustules, nodules, or purpura seen in miliary TB from hematogenous spread; and 4) persistent nodules of the posterior lower calf representing a lobular panniculitis known as *erythema induratum*, a form of a tuberculid. These cutaneous manifestations of TB, along with the many other specific and nonspecific findings, should prompt testing including skin biopsy, tissue culture, screening with blood testing if available such as QuantiFERON-Gold, tuberculin skin testing, and in some, a chest x-ray.

Atypical mycobacterial infections can occur in immunocompetent hosts after trauma, surgery, or exposures to organisms in specific locations such as fish tanks (*Mycobacterium marinum*) or pedicure spas (*Mycobacterium fortuitum*). Immunocompromised individuals are at risk of developing infections with atypical mycobacteria such as the *Mycobacterium avium-intracellulare* as seen in patients infected with HIV. Despite the great variety of atypical mycobacterial organisms, the clinical findings tend to be similar and nonspecific, including papules, pustules, nodules, and ulcers. They can be localized or widespread depending on the cause, exposure, and underlying immune status of the patient. Tissue culture with antibiotic sensitivity testing is helpful, but can take several weeks to be completed.

This chapter of the atlas catalogs the many cutaneous findings seen in patients with both TB and nontuberculous mycobacterial infections.

Fig. 16.1 Primary inoculation tuberculosis.

Fig. 16.2 Tuberculosis verrucosa cutis. *Courtesy Scott Norton, MD.*

Fig. 16.3 Tuberculosis verrucosa cutis.

Fig. 16.4 Tuberculosis verrucosa cutis. *Courtesy Shyam Verma, MBBS, DVD.*

Fig. 16.5 Tuberculosis verrucosa cutis. *Courtesy Debabrata Bandyopadhyay, MD.*

Fig. 16.6 Lupus vulgaris. *Courtesy Debabrata Bandyopadhyay, MD.*

Fig. 16.7 Lupus vulgaris. *Courtesy Debabrata Bandyopadhyay.*

Fig. 16.8 Lupus vulgaris. *Courtesy Steven Binnick, MD.*

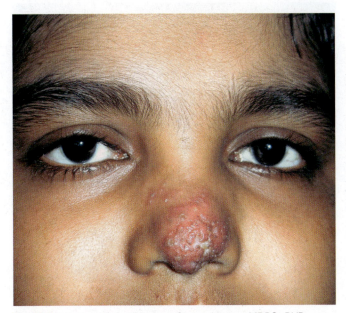

Fig. 16.9 Lupus vulgaris. *Courtesy Shyam Verma, MBBS, DVD.*

Fig. 16.10 Lupus vulgaris. *Courtesy Debabrata Bandyopadhyay, MD.*

Fig. 16.11 Lupus vulgaris. *Courtesy Debabrata Bandyopadhyay, MD.*

Fig. 16.12 Scrofuloderma. *Courtesy James Steger, MD.*

Fig. 16.13 Scrofuloderma. *Courtesy Steven Binnick, MD.*

Fig. 16.14 Scrofuloderma.

Fig. 16.15 Scrofuloderma. *Courtesy Scott Norton, MD.*

Fig. 16.16 Linear scarring after scrofuloderma.

Fig. 16.17 Metastatic tuberculosis. *Courtesy Debabrata Bandyopadhyay, MD.*

Fig. 16.18 Papulonecrotic tuberculid. *Courtesy James Steger, MD.*

Fig. 16.19 Erythema induratum.

Fig. 16.20 *Mycobacterium marinum* in an immunocompromised patient.

Fig. 16.21 Mycobacterium marinum infection. Courtesy Steven Binnick, MD.

Fig. 16.22 Mycobacterium marinum infection. Courtesy Steven Binnick, MD.

Fig. 16.23 Mycobacterium marinum infection. Courtesy Edward C. Oldfield, III, MD.

Fig. 16.24 Mycobacterium marinum infection in a sporotrichoid pattern. Courtesy Dr. Tan Hiok Hee.

Fig. 16.25 *Mycobacterium marinum* infection in a sporotrichoid pattern.

Fig. 16.26 *Mycobacterium marinum* infection in a sporotrichoid pattern.

Fig. 16.27 Disseminated *Mycobacterium marinum* infection in a lupus patient. Minocycline pigmentation is present. *Courtesy Curt Samlaska, MD.*

Fig. 16.28 Buruli ulcer. *Courtesy Scott Norton, MD.*

Fig. 16.29 *Mycobacterium haemophilum* cellulitis and ulcer. *Courtesy Dr. Ang Chia Chun.*

Fig. 16.30 *Mycobacterium fortuitum* infection.

Fig. 16.31 *Mycobacterium fortuitum* infection.

Fig. 16.32 *Mycobacterium chelonae* infection in a patient with chronic obstructive pulmonary disease on prednisone.

Fig. 16.33 *Mycobacterium chelonae* infection in a lung transplant patient.

Fig. 16.34 *Mycobacterium abscessus* infection in an otherwise healthy patient.

Fig. 16.35 *Mycobacterium chelonae* infection. Courtesy Edward C. Oldfield, III, MD.

Fig. 16.36 Generalized *Mycobacterium avium-intracellulare* infection in an HIV-infected patient. Courtesy Curt Samlaska, MD.

Fig. 16.37 Generalized *Mycobacterium avium-intracellulare* infection in an HIV-infected patient. Courtesy Curt Samlaska, MD.

Fig. 16.38 Cutaneous *Mycobacterium avium-intracellulare* infection.

Fig. 16.39 Cutaneous *Mycobacterium kansasii* infection.

Hansen Disease 17

Clinical manifestations of leprosy vary from the subtle hypopigmented patches of indeterminate leprosy to the diffuse facial infiltration and nodules of lepromatous leprosy. The clinical and histologic manifestations of the disease are a reflection of the immune response and bacterial burden. Indeterminate leprosy demonstrates sparse perivascular lymphoid infiltrates and onion skin fibrosis as a manifestation of chronicity. The clinical findings are also subtle with little to no erythema or induration. Tuberculoid leprosy presents as indurated erythematous anesthetic plaques; borderline disease is characterized by annular erythematous indurated lesions, and the lepromatous pole by papules, nodules, and diffuse induration with loss of lateral eyebrows and progression to leonine facies. Diffuse induration correlates with a diffuse dermal histiocytic infiltrate. Globi (clusters of organisms) are easily identified in tissue sections.

Reactional states include reversal reactions characterized by increasing induration, pain, and neurologic manifestations as a reflection of a heightened cell-mediated immune response. In contrast, erythema nodosum leprosum represents a reaction to locally formed immune complexes and is characterized histologically by leukocytoclastic vasculitis in areas of high bacterial burden. Lucio phenomenon demonstrates thrombosis of large and small vessels with variable vasculitis and presents with stellate ulcers and retiform purpura on a background of indurated skin. This portion of the atlas will guide you through the various clinical presentations of Hansen disease.

Fig. 17.2 Indeterminate leprosy.

Fig. 17.1 Indeterminate leprosy. *Courtesy Shyam Verma, MBBS, DVD.*

Fig. 17.3 Early tuberculoid leprosy. *Courtesy Shyam Verma, MBBS, DVD.*

Fig. 17.4 Tuberculoid leprosy.

Fig. 17.5 Tuberculoid leprosy. *Courtesy Steven Binnick, MD.*

Fig. 17.6 Tuberculoid leprosy.

Fig. 17.7 Tuberculoid leprosy. *Courtesy Dermatology Division, University of Campinas, Brazil.*

Fig. 17.8 Greater auricular nerve enlargement in leprosy. *Courtesy Dermatology Division, University of Campinas, Brazil.*

Fig. 17.9 Nerve enlargement in leprosy. *Courtesy Debabrata Bandyopadhyay.*

Fig. 17.10 Borderline tuberculoid leprosy. *Courtesy Shyam Verma, MBBS, DVD.*

Fig. 17.11 Borderline tuberculoid leprosy.

Fig. 17.12 Borderline tuberculoid leprosy.

Fig. 17.13 Borderline tuberculoid leprosy.

Fig. 17.14 Borderline tuberculoid leprosy.

Fig. 17.15 Borderline tuberculoid leprosy. *Courtesy Shyam Verma, MBBS, DVD.*

Fig. 17.16 Borderline leprosy. *Courtesy Shyam Verma, MBBS, DVD.*

Fig. 17.17 Borderline leprosy. *Courtesy Shyam Verma, MBBS, DVD.*

Fig. 17.18 Borderline lepromatous leprosy.

Fig. 17.19 Borderline lepromatous leprosy.

Fig. 17.20 Borderline lepromatous leprosy. *Courtesy Curt Samlaska, MD.*

Fig. 17.21 Borderline lepromatous leprosy. *Courtesy Curt Samlaska, MD.*

Fig. 17.22 Borderline lepromatous leprosy. *Courtesy Curt Samlaska, MD.*

Fig. 17.23 Lepromatous leprosy. *Courtesy Michelle Weir, MD.*

Fig. 17.24 Lepromatous leprosy. *Courtesy Tatiana C. P. Cordeiro de Andrade, MD.*

Fig. 17.25 Lepromatous leprosy. *Courtesy Tatiana C. P. Cordeiro de Andrade, MD.*

Fig. 17.26 Lepromatous leprosy. *Courtesy Shyam Verma, MBBS, DVD.*

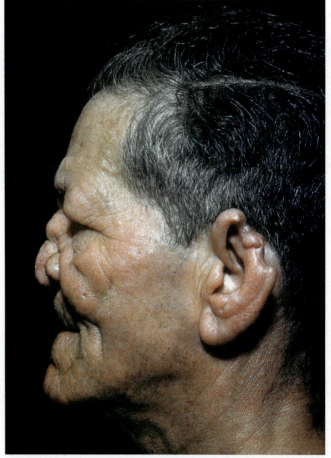

Fig. 17.27 Lepromatous leprosy. *Courtesy Steven Binnick, MD.*

Fig. 17.28 Lepromatous leprosy.

Fig. 17.29 Diffuse leprosy of Lucio. Note loss of eyebrows.

Fig. 17.30 Histiocytoid leprosy.

Fig. 17.31 Histiocytoid leprosy. *Courtesy James Steger, MD.*

Fig. 17.32 Secondary changes due to neurologic disease in leprosy.

Fig. 17.33 Secondary changes due to neurologic disease in leprosy.

Fig. 17.34 Neuropathic ulcer in leprosy. *Courtesy Shyam Verma, MBBS, DVD.*

Fig. 17.35 Neuropathic ulcer in leprosy. *Courtesy Shyam Verma, MBBS, DVD.*

Fig. 17.36 Ichthyosis and pigmentation after clofazimine in leprosy. *Courtesy Scott Norton, MD.*

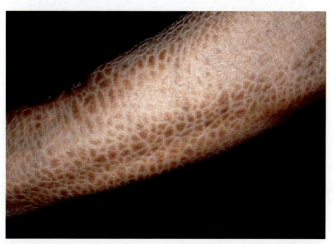

Fig. 17.37 Acquired ichthyosis in leprosy. *Courtesy Scott Norton, MD.*

Fig. 17.38 Type 1 reactional leprosy. *Courtesy Lauro de Souza Lima Institute, Brazil.*

Fig. 17.39 Type 1 reactional leprosy. *Courtesy Lauro de Souza Lima Institute, Brazil.*

Fig. 17.40 Type 1 reactional leprosy. *Courtesy Shyam Verma, MBBS, DVD.*

Fig. 17.41 Type 1 reactional leprosy. *Courtesy Lauro de Souza Lima Institute, Brazil.*

Fig. 17.42 Erythema nodosum leprosum reactional leprosy. *Courtesy Adela Cardones, MD.*

Fig. 17.43 Type 2 reactional leprosy. *Courtesy Lauro de Souza Lima Institute, Brazil.*

Fig. 17.44 Type 2 reactional leprosy. *Courtesy Lauro de Souza Lima Institute, Brazil.*

Fig. 17.45 Type 2 reactional leprosy. *Courtesy Aileen Chang, MD.*

Fig. 17.46 Lucio phenomenon. *Courtesy Lauro de Souza Lima Institute, Brazil.*

Fig. 17.47 Lucio phenomenon. *Courtesy Lauro de Souza Lima Institute, Brazil.*

Syphilis, Yaws, Bejel, and Pinta 18

Syphilis has been dubbed "the great imitator" for its ability to assume varied morphologies. Primary syphilis is characterized by a chancre—a minimally tender, indurated ulcer—or less commonly by syphilitic balanoposthitis. Secondary syphilis can present with indurated, ham- to copper-colored papulosquamous lesions with peripheral adherent scale, annular and gyrate lesions, patchy alopecia, and gray indurated mucous patches. The palms and soles may be involved. Tertiary syphilis is characterized by destructive granulomatous disease that often involves the central face, causing destruction of the nasal bridge. Congenital syphilis can present with periostitis leading to saber shins and frontal bossing, mucositis, and gray fissured periorificial mucous patches. Vesiculobullous lesions may be seen in congenital syphilis. Pustular and crusted lesions characterize lues maligna and rupioid syphilis, respectively.

A high index of suspicion is required, and serologic testing can be falsely negative (prozone reaction) as a result of very high antibody titers. Recognition of morphologies suggestive of syphilis should prompt appropriate testing to include a skin biopsy.

Fig. 18.2 Primary syphilis.

Fig. 18.1 Primary syphilis.

Fig. 18.3 Primary syphilis.

Fig. 18.4 Primary syphilis.

Fig. 18.5 Primary syphilis.

Fig. 18.6 Primary syphilis.

Fig. 18.7 Primary syphilis.

Fig. 18.8 Primary syphilis.

Fig. 18.9 Primary syphilis; chancre is on patient's left palate.

Fig. 18.10 Healing primary syphilis on upper lip; concomitant mucous patch of secondary syphilis on tongue.

Fig. 18.11 Primary syphilis.

Fig. 18.12 Primary syphilis with secondary lesions on the palms.

Fig. 18.13 Secondary syphilis.

Fig. 18.14 Secondary syphilis.

Fig. 18.15 Secondary syphilis.

Fig. 18.16 Secondary syphilis.

Fig. 18.17 Secondary syphilis.

Fig. 18.18 Secondary syphilis.

Fig. 18.19 Secondary syphilis.

Fig. 18.20 Secondary syphilis.

Fig. 18.21 Secondary syphilis and Kaposi sarcoma (on the right arm) of this HIV-infected patient.

Fig. 18.22 Secondary syphilis in an HIV-infected patient. *Courtesy Scott Norton, MD.*

Fig. 18.23 Secondary syphilis.

Fig. 18.24 Secondary syphilis.

Fig. 18.25 Secondary syphilis.

Fig. 18.26 Secondary syphilis.

Fig. 18.27 Secondary syphilis.

Fig. 18.28 Mucous patch of the tongue.

Fig. 18.29 Secondary syphilis, mucous patch. *Courtesy Steven Binnick, MD.*

Fig. 18.30 Secondary syphilis, mucous patch.

Fig. 18.31 Condyloma lata.

Fig. 18.32 Condyloma lata.

Fig. 18.33 Condyloma lata. *Courtesy Ken Greer, MD.*

Fig. 18.34 Condyloma lata.

Fig. 18.35 Secondary syphilis alopecia.

Fig. 18.36 Secondary syphilis alopecia.

Fig. 18.37 Secondary syphilis alopecia.

Fig. 18.38 Tertiary syphilis.

Fig. 18.39 Tertiary syphilis. *Courtesy Lauro de Souza Lima Institute, Brazil.*

Fig. 18.40 Tertiary syphilis. *Courtesy Lauro de Souza Lima Institute, Brazil.*

Fig. 18.41 Congenital syphilis. *Courtesy Paul Honig, MD.*

Fig. 18.42 Congenital syphilis. *Courtesy Paul Honig, MD.*

Fig. 18.43 Congenital syphilis with Hutchinson teeth.

Fig. 18.44 Congenital syphilis with mulberry molar.

Fig. 18.45 Congenital syphilis.

Fig. 18.46 Congenital syphilis, scars from rhagades.

Fig. 18.47 Yaws.

Fig. 18.48 Yaws.

Fig. 18.49 Yaws.

Fig. 18.50 Yaws.

Fig. 18.51 Bejel. *Courtesy Steven Binnick, MD.*

Fig. 18.52 Pinta. *Courtesy Steven Binnick, MD.*

Fig. 18.53 Pinta. *Courtesy Steven Binnick, MD.*

Viral Diseases 19

Viral diseases can manifest as nonspecific exanthems, such as in measles and many other morbilliform eruptions, or more specific patterned eruptions, such as the papules on the cheeks, elbows, knees, and buttocks seen in Gianotti-Crosti syndrome. Primary lesions of viral infections vary from the vesicles seen in many herpetic and enteroviral conditions to the petechiae seen in the papular-purpuric gloves-and-socks syndrome due to parvovirus B19.

Skin lesion distribution is helpful when distinguishing between common vesicular eruptions, including the grouped localized vesicles and erosions seen in herpes simplex virus, compared with the dermatomal vesicular eruptions secondary to herpes zoster virus. As with other infections, the patient's underlying immune status also plays a role in the clinical findings, as evidenced by the verrucous herpetic lesions or severe disseminated herpes zoster seen in immunocompromised patients. Other underlying conditions, such as concurrent eczema, can also contribute to the patterns of involvement as seen in eczema herpeticum and the newly coined *eczema coxsackium* due to Coxsackie virus A6. Obtaining viral cultures and polymerase chain reaction specimens from these lesions is a common way to establish the exact cause of many vesicular viral eruptions.

The age of the patient can particularly affect the cutaneous manifestations of viral illnesses, including the extramedullary hematopoiesis presenting as purple nodules in congenital cytomegalovirus infections ("blueberry muffin baby") or the classic "slapped cheek" appearance due to erythema infectiosum (parvovirus B19) seen most commonly in school-aged children.

Uncommon viral infections are included, such as the zoonotic poxviruses like Orf that cause self-limited papulonodules, as well as even more exotic arthropod-borne viral infections such as Dengue and Chikungunya virus. Common viral conditions are included here as well, such as the dome-shaped, umbilicated, shiny papules of molluscum contagiosum and verruca vulgaris in its many forms secondary to human papillomavirus.

Finally, amid the many viral illnesses included in this portion of the atlas, human immunodeficiency virus deserves particular mention because it can cause a polymorphous primary eruption in the skin and is also associated with many other coinfections such as human herpesvirus 8 in the form of Kaposi sarcoma.

This portion of the atlas highlights the vast range of skin manifestations produced by viral illnesses.

Fig. 19.1 Primary herpes simplex infection.

Fig. 19.2 Primary herpes simplex infection.

Fig. 19.3 Primary herpes simplex infection.

Fig. 19.4 Recurrent herpes simplex infection.

Fig. 19.5 Recurrent herpes simplex infection. *Courtesy Steven Binnick, MD.*

Fig. 19.6 Recurrent herpes simplex infection. *Courtesy Steven Binnick, MD.*

Fig. 19.7 Recurrent herpes simplex infection.

Fig. 19.8 Recurrent herpes simplex infection. *Courtesy Steven Binnick, MD.*

Fig. 19.9 Recurrent herpes simplex infection. *Courtesy Steven Binnick, MD.*

Fig. 19.10 Herpetic sycosis.

Fig. 19.11 Herpetic sycosis.

Fig. 19.12 Herpes gladiatorum.

Fig. 19.13 Herpes gladiatorum.

Fig. 19.14 Herpetic whitlow. *Courtesy Steven Binnick, MD.*

Fig. 19.15 Herpetic infection of the palm.

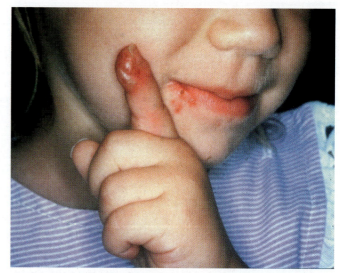

Fig. 19.16 Autoinoculation recurrent labial herpes of the finger.

Fig. 19.17 Herpes genitalis. *Courtesy Steven Binnick, MD.*

Fig. 19.18 Herpes genitalis. *Courtesy Steven Binnick, MD.*

Fig. 19.19 Herpes genitalis. *Courtesy Steven Binnick, MD.*

Fig. 19.20 Recurrent herpes simplex buttock.

Fig. 19.21 Intrauterine herpes simplex infection.

Fig. 19.22 Eczema herpeticum.

Fig. 19.23 Eczema herpeticum.

Fig. 19.24 Eczema herpeticum.

Fig. 19.25 Disseminated herpes simplex infection.

Fig. 19.26 Disseminated herpes simplex infection.

Fig. 19.27 Ulcerative herpes simplex in an HIV-infected patient.

Fig. 19.28 Ulcerative herpes simplex in an HIV-infected patient.

Fig. 19.29 Crusted ulcerative herpes simplex in an HIV-infected patient.

Fig. 19.30 Varicella.

Fig. 19.31 Varicella.

Fig. 19.32 Varicella.

Fig. 19.33 Varicella. *Courtesy Steven Binnick, MD.*

Fig. 19.34 Herpes zoster.

Fig. 19.35 Herpes zoster.

Fig. 19.36 Herpes zoster. *Courtesy Steven Binnick, MD.*

Fig. 19.37 Herpes zoster with Ramsay Hunt syndrome. *Courtesy Steven Binnick, MD.*

Fig. 19.38 Herpes zoster. *Courtesy Steven Binnick, MD.*

Fig. 19.39 Herpes zoster.

Fig. 19.40 Herpes zoster.

Fig. 19.41 Herpes zoster scarring. *Courtesy Steven Binnick, MD.*

Fig. 19.42 Herpes zoster.

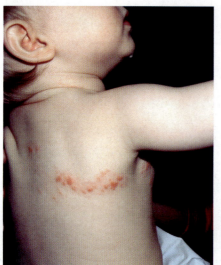

Fig. 19.43 Herpes zoster in an 11-month-old patient.

Fig. 19.44 Herpes zoster, prevesicular.

Fig. 19.45 Herpes zoster in a Hodgkin disease patient.

Fig. 19.46 Herpes zoster in an HIV-infected patient.

Fig. 19.47 Mononucleosis. *Courtesy Steven Binnick, MD.*

Fig. 19.48 Oral hairy leukoplakia.

Fig. 19.49 Oral hairy leukoplakia.

Fig. 19.50 Cytomegaloviral infection in a newborn. *Courtesy Paul Honig, MD.*

Fig. 19.51 Cytomegaloviral ulcer in an HIV-infected patient.

Fig. 19.53 Kaposi sarcoma in an HIV-infected patient.

Fig. 19.55 Necrolytic acral erythema. *Courtesy Carrie Kovarik, MD.*

Fig. 19.52 Kaposi sarcoma in an HIV-infected patient.

Fig. 19.54 Kaposi sarcoma in an HIV-infected patient.

Fig. 19.56 Necrolytic acral erythema. *Courtesy Scott Norton, MD.*

Fig. 19.57 Necrolytic acral erythema. First published in Hivnor CM, Yan AC, Junkins-Hopkins JM, Honig PJ: Nercrolytic acral erythema. J Am Acad Dermatol 2004: 50: S121-124.

Fig. 19.58 Necrolytic acral erythema. First published in Hivnor CM, Yan AC, Junkins-Hopkins JM, Honig PJ: Nercrolytic acral erythema. J Am Acad Dermatol 2004: 50: S121-124.

Fig. 19.59 Necrolytic acral erythema.

Fig. 19.60 Gianotti-Crosti syndrome. *Courtesy Curt Samlaska, MD.*

Fig. 19.61 Gianotti-Crosti syndrome.

Fig. 19.62 Gianotti-Crosti syndrome. *Courtesy Curt Samlaska, MD.*

Fig. 19.63 Smallpox scarring. *Courtesy Steven Binnick, MD.*

Fig. 19.64 Vaccinia vaccination with autoinoculation.

Fig. 19.65 Vaccinia vaccination site with reactive erythema.

Fig. 19.66 Disseminated vaccinia.

Fig. 19.67 Orf.

Fig. 19.68 Milker nodule.

Fig. 19.69 Molluscum contagiosum. *Courtesy Steven Binnick, MD.*

Fig. 19.70 Molluscum contagiosum. *Courtesy Steven Binnick, MD.*

Fig. 19.71 Molluscum contagiosum.

Fig. 19.72 Molluscum contagiosum.

Fig. 19.73 Giant molluscum contagiosum.

Fig. 19.74 Molluscum contagiosum.

Fig. 19.75 Giant molluscum contagiosum. *Courtesy Shyam Verma, MBBS, DVD.*

Fig. 19.76 Molluscum contagiosum in an HIV-infected patient.

Fig. 19.77 Molluscum dermatitis.

Fig. 19.78 Herpangina.

Fig. 19.79 Hand-foot-and-mouth disease.

Fig. 19.80 Hand-foot-and-mouth disease.

Fig. 19.81 Hand-foot-and-mouth disease. *Courtesy Steven Binnick, MD.*

Fig. 19.82 Hand-foot-and-mouth disease. *Courtesy Steven Binnick, MD.*

Fig. 19.83 Coxsackie A6 hand-foot-and-mouth disease.

Fig. 19.84 Coxsackie A6 hand-foot-and-mouth disease.

Fig. 19.85 Coxsackie A6 hand-foot-and-mouth disease. *Courtesy Scott Norton, MD.*

Fig. 19.86 Rubeola (measles).

Fig. 19.87 Rubeola (measles).

Fig. 19.88 Rubeola (measles) in a photodistribution.

Fig. 19.89 Koplik spots.

Fig. 19.90 Rubella.

Fig. 19.91 Forschheimer spots in rubella.

Fig. 19.92 Asymmetric periflexural exanthem of childhood.

Fig. 19.93 Asymmetric periflexural exanthem of childhood. *Courtesy Steven Binnick, MD.*

Fig. 19.94 Erythema infectiosum.

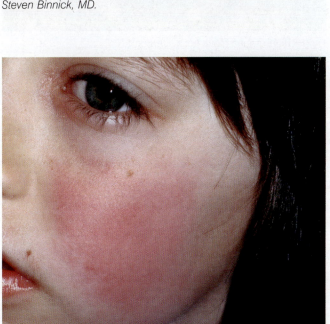

Fig. 19.95 Erythema infectiosum. *Courtesy Steven Binnick, MD.*

Fig. 19.96 Erythema infectiosum. *Courtesy Steven Binnick, MD.*

Fig. 19.97 Erythema infectiosum.

Fig. 19.98 Erythema infectiosum. *Courtesy Curt Samlaska, MD.*

Fig. 19.99 Purpuric glove-sock syndrome.

Fig. 19.100 Purpuric glove-sock syndrome.

Fig. 19.101 Dengue fever.

Fig. 19.102 Dengue fever.

Fig. 19.103 Dengue fever.

Fig. 19.104 Chikungunya fever. *Courtesy Warren R. Heymann, MD.*

Fig. 19.105 Warts. *Courtesy Steven Binnick, MD.*

Fig. 19.106 Warts. *Courtesy Steven Binnick, MD.*

Fig. 19.107 Warts.

Fig. 19.108 Flat warts.

Fig. 19.109 Warts.

Fig. 19.110 Warts. *Courtesy Scott Norton, MD.*

Fig. 19.111 Periungual warts. *Courtesy Steven Binnick, MD.*

Fig. 19.112 Subungual wart. *Courtesy Curt Samlaska, MD.*

Fig. 19.113 Plantar warts.

Fig. 19.114 Plantar warts.

Fig. 19.115 Extensive warts in a patient with gastrointestinal lymphangiomatosis.

Fig. 19.116 Extensive warts as seen in immunodeficiencies such as WHIM and DOCK8.

Fig. 19.117 Condylomata acuminata. *Courtesy Steven Binnick, MD.*

Fig. 19.118 Condylomata acuminata. *Courtesy Steven Binnick, MD.*

Fig. 19.119 Condylomata acuminata. *Courtesy Steven Binnick, MD.*

Fig. 19.120 Condylomata acuminata. *Courtesy Steven Binnick, MD.*

Fig. 19.121 Condylomata acuminata.

Fig. 19.122 Bowenoid papulosis.

Fig. 19.123 Bowenoid papulosis. *Courtesy Steven Binnick, MD.*

Fig. 19.124 Buschke-Lowenstein tumor. *Courtesy Shyam Verma, MBBS, DVD.*

Fig. 19.125 Genital warts in a child.

Fig. 19.126 Oral wart.

Fig. 19.127 Oral wart.

Fig. 19.128 Myrmecia.

Fig. 19.129 Epidermodysplasia verruciformis in an HIV-infected patient.

Fig. 19.130 Epidermodysplasia verruciformis in an HIV-infected patient.

Fig. 19.131 Trichodysplasia spinulosa. *Courtesy Kari Wanat, MD.*

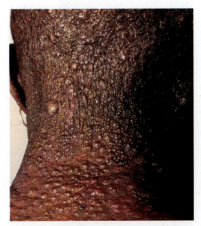

Fig. 19.132 HTLV-1 dermatosis. *Courtesy Alain Rook, MD.*

Fig. 19.133 HTLV-1 dermatosis. *Courtesy Robert Micheletti, MD.*

Fig. 19.134 Primary HIV infection.

Fig. 19.135 Thrush in an HIV-infected patient. *Courtesy Steven Binnick, MD.*

Fig. 19.136 Thrush and resolving chancre in an HIV-infected patient.

Fig. 19.137 Proximal white onychomycosis in an HIV-infected patient.

Fig. 19.138 Herpes simplex and seborrheic dermatitis in an HIV-infected patient.

Fig. 19.139 Chronic herpes simplex in an HIV-infected patient.

Fig. 19.140 Chronic ulcerative herpes simplex in an HIV-infected patient.

Fig. 19.141 Herpes zoster in an HIV-infected patient.

Fig. 19.142 Molluscum contagiosum in an HIV-infected patient.

Fig. 19.143 Condylomata acuminata in an HIV-infected patient.

Fig. 19.144 Condylomata acuminata in an HIV-infected patient.

Fig. 19.145 Epidermodysplasia verruciformis in an HIV-infected patient. *Courtesy Scott Norton, MD.*

Fig. 19.146 Oral hairy leukoplakia in an HIV-infected patient.

Fig. 19.147 Oral Kaposi sarcoma in an HIV-infected patient.

Fig. 19.148 Kaposi sarcoma in an HIV-infected patient.

Fig. 19.149 Kaposi sarcoma in an HIV-infected patient.

Fig. 19.150 Crusted scabies in an HIV-infected patient.

Fig. 19.151 Hair straightening in an HIV-infected patient.

Fig. 19.152 Long eyelashes in an HIV-infected patient.

Fig. 19.153 Acquired ichthyosis in an HIV-infected patient.

Fig. 19.154 Reactive arthritis in an HIV-infected patient.

Fig. 19.155 Eosinophilic folliculitis in an HIV-infected patient.

Fig. 19.156 Eosinophilic folliculitis in an HIV-infected patient.

Parasitic Infestations, Stings, and Bites 20

Bites and infestations present with wide-ranging manifestations, including papules, vesicles, excoriations, and urticarial lesions. Bedbug bites often involve the arms and develop clinical features of prurigo nodularis. A biopsy will demonstrate a wedge-shaped perivascular lymphoid infiltrate with endothelial swelling and eosinophils, suggesting the correct diagnosis.

Cutaneous larva migrans demonstrates an erythematous serpiginous lesion. The worm is located ahead of the advancing border of the lesion, as the cutaneous reaction is a manifestation of a delayed-type immune response to the organism.

Recognition of arthropods of medical importance is critical to allow assessment of the risk of vector-borne disease and guide management. The skin is often affected by ectoparasites as well as endoparasites, and this section of the atlas will provide a guide to identification of the most important organisms.

Fig. 20.1 Old World leishmaniasis.

Fig. 20.2 Old World leishmaniasis.

Fig. 20.3 Old World leishmaniasis.

Fig. 20.4 New World leishmaniasis.

Fig. 20.5 New World leishmaniasis.

Fig. 20.6 New World leishmaniasis.

Fig. 20.7 New World leishmaniasis.

Fig. 20.8 New World leishmaniasis. *Courtesy Scott Norton, MD.*

Fig. 20.10 New World leishmaniasis.

Fig. 20.9 New World leishmaniasis.

Fig. 20.11 New World leishmaniasis.

Fig. 20.12 Mucocutaneous leishmaniasis, same patient as Fig. 20.11.

Fig. 20.13 Mucocutaneous leishmaniasis.

Fig. 20.14 Mucocutaneous leishmaniasis.

Fig. 20.15 Mucocutaneous leishmaniasis. *Courtesy Lauro de Souza Lima Institute, Brazil.*

Fig. 20.16 Anergic leishmaniasis.

Fig. 20.17 Anergic leishmaniasis. *Courtesy Lauro de Souza Lima Institute, Brazil.*

Fig. 20.18 Anergic leishmaniasis.

Fig. 20.19 Post-kala-azar dermal leishmaniasis. *Courtesy Debabrata Bandyopadhyay, MD.*

Fig. 20.20 Triatome bite.

Fig. 20.21 Romana sign, Chagas disease.

Fig. 20.22 Toxoplasmosis. Note erythema of eyelids. *Courtesy Steven Binnick, MD.*

Fig. 20.23 Portuguese man of war dermatitis. *Courtesy Rui Tavares Bello, MD.*

Fig. 20.24 Jellyfish dermatitis. *Courtesy Steven Binnick, MD.*

Fig. 20.25 Sea wasp dermatitis. *Courtesy Curt Samlaska, MD.*

Fig. 20.26 Healed jellyfish dermatitis. *Courtesy Steven Binnick, MD.*

Fig. 20.27 Seabather eruption. *Courtesy Scott Norton, MD.*

Fig. 20.28 Fire coral dermatitis. *Courtesy Steven Binnick, MD.*

Fig. 20.29 Coral granuloma.

Fig. 20.30 Sea urchin injury. *Courtesy Scott Norton, MD.*

Fig. 20.31 Sea urchin granuloma. *Courtesy Steven Binnick, MD.*

Fig. 20.32 Seaweed dermatitis. *Courtesy Curt Samlaska, MD.*

Fig. 20.33 Swimmer itch. *Courtesy Camille Introcaso, MD.*

Fig. 20.34 Katayama fever–associated dermatitis. *Courtesy Scott Norton, MD.*

Fig. 20.35 Cutaneous larva migrans.

Fig. 20.36 Cutaneous larva migrans.

Fig. 20.37 Cutaneous larva migrans.

Fig. 20.38 Cutaneous larva migrans. *Courtesy Steven Binnick, MD.*

Fig. 20.39 Gnathostomiasis. *Courtesy Scott Norton, MD.*

Fig. 20.40 Filariasis. *Courtesy Scott Norton, MD.*

Fig. 20.41 Filariasis.

Fig. 20.42 Filariasis.

Fig. 20.43 Calabar swelling. *Courtesy Curt Samlaska, MD.*

Fig. 20.44 Loiasis; worm is in patient's left upper eyelid. *Courtesy Curt Samlaska, MD.*

Fig. 20.45 Onchocerciasis with acute papular eruption.

Fig. 20.46 Onchocerciasis with peau d'orange edema.

Fig. 20.47 Onchocerciasis with papules and dyspigmentation. *Courtesy Scott Norton, MD.*

Fig. 20.48 Onchocerciasis with dyspigmentation. *Courtesy Scott Norton, MD.*

Fig. 20.49 Onchocercoma.

Fig. 20.50 Onchocerciasis with hanging groin.

Fig. 20.51 Insect bite.

Fig. 20.52 Insect bites.

Fig. 20.53 Bedbug bites.

Fig. 20.54 Bedbug bites.

Fig. 20.55 Pediculosis capitis.

Fig. 20.56 Pediculosis capitis.

Fig. 20.57 Pediculosis corporis.

Fig. 20.58 Pediculosis; nits in clothing.

Fig. 20.59 Pediculosis pubis.

Fig. 20.60 Maculae ceruleae.

Fig. 20.61 Pubic lice on the eyelashes.

Fig. 20.62 Myiasis. *Courtesy Steven Binnick, MD.*

Fig. 20.63 Myiasis.

Fig. 20.64 Extraction of larva after treating with petrolatum.

Fig. 20.65 Paederus (beetle) dermatitis. *Courtesy Shyam Verma, MBBS, DVD.*

Fig. 20.66 Wasp sting.

Fig. 20.67 Bee sting. *Courtesy Steven Binnick, MD.*

Fig. 20.68 Fire ant stings.

Fig. 20.69 Flea bites. *Courtesy Curt Samlaska, MD.*

Fig. 20.70 Flea bites.

Fig. 20.71 Tungiasis. *Courtesy Catherine Quirk, MD.*

Fig. 20.72 Tick bite.

Fig. 20.73 Tick bite site.

Fig. 20.74 Scabies.

Fig. 20.75 Scabies.

Fig. 20.76 Scabies.

Fig. 20.77 Scabies. *Courtesy Shyam Verma, MBBS, DVD.*

Fig. 20.78 Scabies. *Courtesy Shyam Verma, MBBS, DVD.*

Fig. 20.79 Nodular scabies.

Fig. 20.80 Nodular scabies.

Fig. 20.81 Scabies.

Fig. 20.82 Scabies.

Fig. 20.83 Scabies.

Fig. 20.84 Scabies.

Fig. 20.85 Scabies.

Fig. 20.86 Scabies.

Fig. 20.87 Scabies.

Fig. 20.88 Crusted scabies in an HIV-infected patient.

Fig. 20.89 Crusted scabies in an HIV-infected patient. *Courtesy Curt Samlaska, MD.*

Fig. 20.90 Crusted scabies in an HIV-infected patient.

Fig. 20.91 Cheyletiella mite bites. *Courtesy Scott Norton, MD.*

Fig. 20.92 Chigger bites.

Fig. 20.93 Brown recluse spider bite. *Courtesy Steven Binnick, MD.*

Fig. 20.94 Brown recluse spider bite.

Fig. 20.95 Spider bite.

Fig. 20.96 Snake bite.

Fig. 20.97 Russell pit viper bite. *Courtesy Scott Norton, MD.*

Chronic Blistering Dermatoses 21

Immunobullous dermatoses may present with urticarial lesions, blisters, erosions, or pustules. IgA-mediated disease is characterized by annular lesions with a "string of pearls" morphology—bullous in the case of linear IgA bullous dermatosis and pustular or erosive in the case of IgA pemphigus. Pemphigoid typically presents with tense blisters forming on erythematous patches or urticarial plaques. Pemphigus vulgaris often initially appears with oral erosions, but can progress to widely denuded areas of skin. In contrast, pemphigus foliaceus presents with superficial erosions and adherent crusts that resemble macerated cornflakes allowed to dry at the bottom of the bowl. Pemphigus vegetans is characterized by localized, moist, heaped-up crusts, sometimes studded with pustules. Dermatitis herpetiformis presents with intense itching with excoriation and erosions clustered on the posterior scalp, extensor surfaces, and buttocks. Itching is intense, so it is rare to identify intact blisters. This portion of the atlas will guide you through the various clinical presentations of bullous disorders of the skin.

Fig. 21.1 Pemphigus vulgaris. *Courtesy Curt Samlaska, MD.*

Fig. 21.2 Pemphigus vulgaris.

Fig. 21.3 Pemphigus vulgaris with hyperpigmentation.

Fig. 21.4 Pemphigus vulgaris.

Fig. 21.5 Pemphigus vulgaris after radiation therapy.

Fig. 21.6 Oral pemphigus vulgaris. *Courtesy Steven Binnick, MD.*

Fig. 21.7 Oral pemphigus vulgaris. *Courtesy Curt Samlaska, MD.*

Fig. 21.8 Oral pemphigus vulgaris.

Fig. 21.9 Oral pemphigus vulgaris.

Fig. 21.10 Scalp pemphigus vulgaris. *Courtesy Curt Samlaska, MD.*

Fig. 21.11 Pemphigus vulgaris. *Courtesy Curt Samlaska, MD.*

Fig. 21.12 Pemphigus vulgaris.

Fig. 21.13 Nail pemphigus vulgaris, paronychia type.

Fig. 21.14 Nail pemphigus vulgaris, onychomadesis type.

Fig. 21.16 Pemphigus vegetans. *Courtesy Steven Binnick, MD.*

Fig. 21.15 Pemphigus vulgaris.

Fig. 21.17 Pemphigus vegetans. *Courtesy John Stanley, MD.*

Fig. 21.18 Pemphigus foliaceus. *Courtesy Steven Binnick, MD.*

Fig. 21.19 Pemphigus foliaceus.

Fig. 21.20 Pemphigus foliaceus.

Fig. 21.21 Pemphigus foliaceus.

Fig. 21.22 Pemphigus foliaceus.

Fig. 21.23 Pemphigus foliaceus. *Courtesy Debabrata Bandyopadhyay.*

Fig. 21.24 Pemphigus foliaceus. *Courtesy Dermatology Division, University of Campinas, Brazil.*

Fig. 21.25 Fogo selvagem. *Courtesy Dermatology Division, University of Campinas, Brazil.*

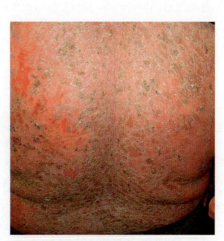

Fig. 21.26 Fogo selvagem. *Courtesy Dermatology Division, University of Campinas, Brazil.*

Fig. 21.27 Pemphigus erythematosus-like pemphigus foliaceus. *Courtesy John Stanley, MD.*

Fig. 21.28 Pemphigus erythematosus. *Courtesy Steven Binnick, MD.*

Fig. 21.29 Paraneoplastic pemphigus. Note enlarged cervical lymph node caused by metastatic tongue cancer. *Courtesy Dermatology Division, University of Campinas, Brazil.*

Fig. 21.30 Paraneoplastic pemphigus.

Fig. 21.31 Intraepidermal neutrophilic IgA dermatosis. *Courtesy John Stanley, MD.*

Fig. 21.32 Intraepidermal neutrophilic IgA dermatosis. *Courtesy John Stanley, MD.*

Fig. 21.33 Intraepidermal neutrophilic IgA dermatosis.

Fig. 21.34 Bullous pemphigoid.

Fig. 21.35 Bullous pemphigoid.

Fig. 21.36 Bullous pemphigoid.

Fig. 21.37 Bullous pemphigoid. *Courtesy Shyam Verma, MBBS, DVD.*

Fig. 21.38 Bullous pemphigoid.

Fig. 21.39 Urticarial bullous pemphigoid.

Fig. 21.40 Urticarial bullous pemphigoid with bullae.

Fig. 21.41 Vesicular bullous pemphigoid. *Courtesy Steven Binnick, MD.*

Fig. 21.42 Infantile bullous pemphigoid.

Fig. 21.43 Erythodermic bullous pemphigoid.

Fig. 21.44 Pemphigoid gestationis.

Fig. 21.45 Pemphigoid gestationis.

Fig. 21.46 Pemphigoid gestationis.

Fig. 21.47 Pemphigoid gestationis. *Courtesy Ken Greer, MD.*

Fig. 21.48 Pruritic urticarial papules and plaques of pregnancy.

Fig. 21.49 Pruritic urticarial papules and plaques of pregnancy.

Fig. 21.50 Cicatricial pemphigoid.

Fig. 21.51 Cicatricial pemphigoid.

Fig. 21.52 Cicatricial pemphigoid. *Courtesy Curt Samlaska, MD.*

Fig. 21.53 Cicatricial pemphigoid. *Courtesy Steven Binnick, MD.*

Fig. 21.54 Brunsting-Perry pemphigoid.

Fig. 21.55 Epidermolysis bullosa acquisita.

Fig. 21.56 Epidermolysis bullosa acquisita.

Fig. 21.57 Epidermolysis bullosa acquisita.

Fig. 21.58 Epidermolysis bullosa acquisita.

Fig. 21.59 Epidermolysis bullosa acquisita.

Fig. 21.60 Inflammatory epidermolysis bullosa acquisita.

Fig. 21.61 Dermatitis herpetiformis. *Courtesy Steven Binnick, MD.*

Fig. 21.62 Dermatitis herpetiformis.

Fig. 21.63 Dermatitis herpetiformis.

Fig. 21.64 Dermatitis herpetiformis.

Fig. 21.65 Urticarial lesions of dermatitis herpetiformis.

Fig. 21.66 Unusual configuration in dermatitis herpetiformis.

Fig. 21.67 Adult linear IgA disease, urticarial type.

Fig. 21.68 Adult linear IgA disease, which is indistinguishable from dermatitis herpetiformis.

Fig. 21.69 Childhood linear IgA disease.

Fig. 21.70 Childhood linear IgA disease.

Fig. 21.71 Childhood linear IgA disease. *Courtesy Paul Honig, MD.*

Fig. 21.72 Childhood linear IgA disease. *Courtesy Debabrata Bandyopadhyay, MD.*

Fig. 21.73 Transient acantholytic dermatosis.

Fig. 21.74 Transient acantholytic dermatosis.

Fig. 21.75 Transient acantholytic dermatosis. *Courtesy Steven Binnick, MD.*

Fig. 21.76 Transient acantholytic dermatosis. *Courtesy Steven Binnick, MD.*

Nutritional Diseases 22

A deficiency or excess of certain required vitamins or minerals can cause specific findings in the skin, hair, nails, and mucosae. This chapter provides images of many of these findings, both common and rare.

Deficiencies in some essential nutrients cause a particular constellation of mucocutaneous and systemic signs and symptoms worth outlining. These include the bleeding gums, corkscrew hairs, easy bruising. and perifollicular hemorrhages seen in the setting of vitamin C deficiency, or scurvy. In pellagra, or vitamin B_3 (niacin) deficiency, a combination of a photodistributed eruption appearing sunburn-like, scaly, hyperpigmented, or atrophic can be seen along with protracted diarrhea, weakness, dementia, paresthesias, and depression. Kwashiorkor, or protein-energy malnutrition, may present with general lightening of the skin and hair, a scaly eruption with superficial peeling of skin resembling flaking paint, and a dermatitis with cracked skin resembling "crazy pavement" in the setting of a patient with signs of edema and poor growth. These nutritional deficiencies can occur due to general malnutrition where food is scarce, but can also occur in individuals with restricted diets or eating disorders (e.g. anorexia nervosa). Lastly, malabsorption states as found in inflammatory bowel diseases can lead to nutritional deficiencies.

Another relatively common deficiency that presents most commonly during infancy is zinc deficiency leading to acrodermatitis enteropathica. In this condition, scaly and erosive patches tend to be well demarcated with heaped-up, sometimes crusted, borders that consistently affect the perioral region, distal extremities, and groin. Affected infants with acrodermatitis enteropathica are notably irritable.

Acrodermatitis enteropathica–like conditions can be seen in some inherited metabolic conditions, including those leading to biotin deficiency.

This portion of the atlas highlights these and other nutrition-related diseases that affect the skin, hair, nails, and mucosal surfaces.

Fig. 22.2 Phrynoderma in a patient with inflammatory bowel disease.

Fig. 22.1 Phrynoderma in a patient with inflammatory bowel disease.

Fig. 22.3 Atrophic tongue as seen in vitamin B deficiencies.

Fig. 22.4 Perléche as seen in vitamin B deficiencies.

Fig. 22.5 Scurvy.

Fig. 22.6 Scurvy.

Fig. 22.7 Scurvy.

Fig. 22.8 Scurvy.

Fig. 22.9 Scurvy.

Fig. 22.10 Scurvy.

Fig. 22.11 Pellagra. *Courtesy Michelle Weir, MD.*

Fig. 22.12 Pellagra. *Courtesy Steven Binnick, MD.*

Fig. 22.13 Pellagra. *Courtesy Shyam Verma, MBBS, DVD.*

Fig. 22.14 Pellagra. *Courtesy Michelle Weir, MD.*

Fig. 22.15 Isoniazid-induced pellagra-like reactions.

Fig. 22.16 Multiple carboxylase deficiency.

Fig. 22.17 Acrodermatitis enteropathica. *Courtesy Paul Honig, MD.*

Fig. 22.18 Acrodermatitis enteropathica.

Fig. 22.19 Acrodermatitis enteropathica.

Fig. 22.20 Acrodermatitis enteropathica.

Fig. 22.21 Acrodermatitis enteropathica.

Fig. 22.22 Acrodermatitis enteropathica. *Courtesy Carrie Kovarik, MD.*

Fig. 22.23 Acrodermatitis enteropathica.

Fig. 22.24 Acrodermatitis enteropathica.

Fig. 22.25 Acrodermatitis enteropathica. *Courtesy Scott Norton, MD.*

Fig. 22.26 Smooth tongue in anemia.

Fig. 22.27 Angular cheilitis as seen in iron deficiency.

Fig. 22.28 Marasmus.

Fig. 22.29 Kwashiorkor. *Courtesy Campbell Stewart, MD.*

Fig. 22.30 Kwashiorkor. *Courtesy Campbell Stewart, MD.*

Fig. 22.31 Kwashiorkor. *Courtesy Campbell Stewart, MD.*

Fig. 22.32 Kwashiorkor.

Fig. 22.33 Kwashiorkor. *Courtesy Carrie Kovarik, MD.*

Fig. 22.34 Kwashiorkor.

Fig. 22.35 Kwashiorkor.

Fig. 22.36 Kwashiorkor.

Fig. 22.37 Kwashiorkor flag sign.

Fig. 22.38 Carotenemia.

Diseases of Subcutaneous Fat   23

Panniculitis presents with deep erythematous nodules, induration, and tenderness. Clinical lesions of erythema nodosum can appear as deep-seated, erythematous, tender nodules or can resemble bruises, giving rise to the term *erythema contusiforme*. The lesions tend to be bilateral except in erythema nodosum migrans, which is generally unilateral and slowly expands to form an annular plaque.

Erythema induratum favors the calves, and ulceration is frequent. Oily fluid often drains from the ulcers. Pancreatic panniculitis presents as indurated plaques, most commonly on the lower legs. The subcutaneous fat elsewhere may also be affected, and multiple areas may be affected. Tenderness of the ankles is commonly reported. Another form of panniculitis is subcutaneous fat necrosis of the newborn, which also presents as hard, indurated areas and demonstrates characteristic intracellular crystalline rosettes histologically.

Lipodermatosclerosis represents ischemic fat necrosis associated with venous stasis. Early lesions present as tender nodules of the lower leg. Over time, the skin becomes erythematous and indurated, with constriction of the lower leg giving the appearance of an inverted champagne bottle. Factitial and infectious panniculitis range in appearance from erythematous nodules to draining indurated plaques, whereas lipodystrophies present with loss of subcutaneous fat, giving a gaunt and muscular appearance. This section of the atlas will focus on the range of cutaneous findings that accompany diseases of the fat.

Fig. 23.2 Erythema nodosum.

Fig. 23.1 Erythema nodosum. *Courtesy Scott Norton, MD.*

Fig. 23.3 Erythema nodosum.

Fig. 23.4 Erythema nodosum.

Fig. 23.5 Erythema nodosum.

Fig. 23.6 Erythema nodosum. *Courtesy Steven Binnick, MD.*

Fig. 23.7 Erythema nodosum.

Fig. 23.8 Chronic erythema nodosum.

Fig. 23.9 Erythema induratum.

Fig. 23.10 Erythema induratum.

Fig. 23.11 Lipodermatosclerosis. *Courtesy Douglas Pugliese, MD.*

Fig. 23.12 Lipodermatosclerosis. *Courtesy Douglas Pugliese, MD.*

Fig. 23.13 Lipodermatosclerosis. *Courtesy Douglas Pugliese, MD.*

Fig. 23.15 Lipodermatosclerosis. *Courtesy Douglas Pugliese, MD.*

Fig. 23.14 Lipodermatosclerosis. *Courtesy Douglas Pugliese, MD.*

Fig. 23.16 Subcutaneous fat necrosis of the newborn.

Fig. 23.17 Subcutaneous fat necrosis of the newborn.

Fig. 23.18 Subcutaneous fat necrosis of the newborn. *Courtesy Scott Norton, MD.*

Fig. 23.19 Subcutaneous fat necrosis of the newborn. *Courtesy Paul Honig, MD.*

Fig. 23.20 Subcutaneous fat necrosis of the newborn.

Fig. 23.21 Cold panniculitis.

Fig. 23.22 Cold panniculitis.

Fig. 23.23 Cold panniculitis from sitting on a cold tractor seat.

Fig. 23.24 Pancreatic panniculitis. *Courtesy Misha Rosenbach, MD.*

Fig. 23.25 Pancreatic panniculitis.

Fig. 23.26 Pancreatic panniculitis. *Courtesy Ken Greer, MD.*

Fig. 23.27 Acquired partial lipodystrophy.

Fig. 23.28 Acquired partial lipodystrophy. *Courtesy Debabrata Bandyopadhyay.*

Fig. 23.29 Acquired partial lipodystrophy.

Fig. 23.30 Acquired partial lipodystrophy.

Fig. 23.31 Annular atrophic panniculitis, inflammatory phase. *Courtesy Marie Wagener, DO and Elise Grgurich, DO.*

Fig. 23.32 Annular atrophic panniculitis, lipoatrophic phase. *Courtesy Marie Wagener, DO and Elise Grgurich, DO.*

Fig. 23.33 Post–steroid injection atrophy.

Fig. 23.34 Post–steroid injection atrophy. *Courtesy Steven Binnick, MD.*

Fig. 23.35 Insulin lipohypertrophy.

Fig. 23.36 Insulin lipohypertrophy.

Endocrine Diseases 24

Endocrine disorders present with a range of findings that may affect any layer of the skin. The associated skin changes can lead the astute physician to suspect the underlying disorder and order appropriate confirmatory tests.

Excess growth hormone before closure of the epiphyses leads to gigantism, whereas in adults it leads to acromegaly with hypertrophy of the chin, nose, and supraorbital ridges and thickening and wrinkling of the forehead, sometimes accompanied by cutis verticis gyrata. The distal digits are expanded. Addison disease leads to generalized hyperpigmentation as well as orolabial pigmented macules and nail streaks, whereas Cushing disease results in moon facies, fat redistribution giving rise to a buffalo hump, and hirsutism. An appreciation of the range of clinical findings in these conditions can lead to the early diagnosis of systemic disease.

Thyroid disease can present with subtle edema, most prominent around the eyes, in the case of hypothyroid myxedema, or with pebbly thickening of the skin of the shins and dorsal foot in Graves disease–associated pretibial myxedema. Necrobiosis lipoidica presents as atrophic, orange-to-yellow plaques with prominent vascularity and occasional ulceration. The plaques often involve the shins. Diabetes can cause acanthosis nigricans, a velvety thickening and darkening of the skin, noted most prominently over the flexures.

Fig. 24.2 Acromegaly.

Fig. 24.1 Acromegalic hand compared with normal.

Fig. 24.3 Acromegaly.

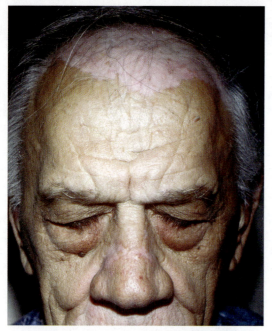

Fig. 24.4 Acromegalic patient with vitiligo. *Courtesy Steven Binnick, MD.*

Fig. 24.5 Enlarged tongue in acromegaly.

Fig. 24.6 Cushing patient with round face, thin hair, hypertrichosis, and acne.

Fig. 24.7 Cushing disease with striae.

Fig. 24.8 Buffalo hump secondary to increased glucocorticoids.

Fig. 24.9 Hypertrichosis in Cushing disease.

Fig. 24.10 Hypertrichosis in Cushing disease.

Fig. 24.11 Skin thinning and ecchymoses in Cushing disease.

Fig. 24.12 Striae in glucocorticoid excess.

Fig. 24.13 Hyperpigmentation in Addison disease. *Courtesy Steven Binnick, MD.*

Fig. 24.14 Hyperpigmentation of chronic traumatic sites in Addison disease. *Courtesy Steven Binnick, MD.*

Fig. 24.15 Hyperpigmentation of the gingiva in Addison disease.

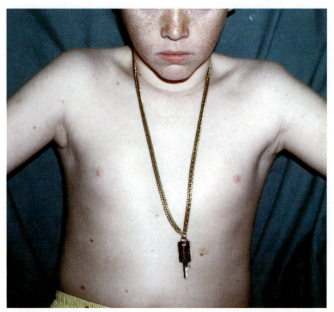

Fig. 24.16 Panhypopituitarism with pale, thin skin.

Fig. 24.17 Panhypopituitarism with pale, thin skin.

Fig. 24.18 Adrenogenital syndrome. *Courtesy Ken Greer, MD.*

Fig. 24.19 Adrenogenital syndrome with ambiguous genitalia. *Courtesy Paul Honig, MD.*

Fig. 24.20 Adrenogenital syndrome. *Courtesy Rui Tavares Bello, MD.*

Fig. 24.21 Adrenogenital syndrome. *Courtesy Rui Tavares Bello, MD.*

Fig. 24.22 Adrenogenital syndrome. *Courtesy Rui Tavares Bello, MD.*

Fig. 24.23 Congenital hypothyroidism.

Fig. 24.24 Congenital hypothyroidism.

Fig. 24.25 Myxedema.

Fig. 24.26 Myxedema.

Fig. 24.27 Puffy, yellow hands in myxedema.

Fig. 24.28 Hair thinning in hypothyroidism.

Fig. 24.29 Dry skin in hypothyroidism.

Fig. 24.30 Palmar keratoderma in hypothyroidism.

Fig. 24.31 Pretibial myxedema.

Fig. 24.32 Pretibial myxedema. *Courtesy Steven Binnick, MD.*

Fig. 24.33 Pretibial myxedema.

Fig. 24.34 Pretibial myxedema.

Fig. 24.35 Pretibial myxedema.

Fig. 24.36 Preradial myxedema.

Fig. 24.37 Thyroid acropachy.

Fig. 24.38 Thyroid acropachy.

Fig. 24.39 Exophthalmos.

Fig. 24.40 Pseudohypoparathyroidism with typical facies. *Courtesy Steven Binnick, MD.*

Fig. 24.41 Pseudohypoparathyroidism.

Fig. 24.42 Pseudohypoparathyroidism.

Fig. 24.43 Multiple endocrine neoplasia type 1 angiofibromas. *Courtesy Thomas Darling, MD, PhD.*

Fig. 24.44 Multiple endocrine neoplasia type 1, collagenomas. *Courtesy Thomas Darling, MD, PhD.*

Fig. 24.45 Acanthosis nigricans.

Fig. 24.46 Acanthosis nigricans. *Courtesy Shyam Verma, MBBS, DVD.*

Fig. 24.47 Acanthosis nigricans.

Fig. 24.48 Acanthosis nigricans.

Fig. 24.49 Axillary granular parakeratosis.

Fig. 24.50 Acanthosis nigricans with malignancy.

Fig. 24.51 Acanthosis nigricans with malignancy.

Fig. 24.52 Acanthosis nigricans with malignancy.

Fig. 24.53 Type B syndrome.

Fig. 24.54 Type B syndrome.

Fig. 24.55 Type B syndrome (close up of acanthosis nigricans on the back).

Fig. 24.56 Type B syndrome.

Fig. 24.57 Tripe palms in type B syndrome.

Abnormalities of Dermal Fibrous and Elastic Tissue

25

This chapter includes a variety of conditions, all resulting from either inherited or acquired changes in the collagen or elastic tissue of the skin.

Some inherited syndromes with particularly unique skin findings include forms of Ehlers-Danlos syndrome (EDS). Affected individuals are noted to have doughy skin that is hyperextensible. Skin is prone to wide "fish-mouth" wounds, molluscoid pseudotumors, and atrophic scars. In contrast, those patients with inherited forms of cutis laxa produce widespread drooping, redundant skin with pendulous folds. Pseudoxanthoma elasticum (PXE) can present with yellowish papules predominantly on the lateral neck said to resemble "plucked chicken skin," as well as lax skin akin to that seen in some forms of cutis laxa. Marfan syndrome is included here due to its underlying genetic mutation in fibrillin-1 that affects connective tissues. In Marfan syndrome characteristic physical findings include tall stature, high-arched palate, and arachnodactyly. Knowledge of the skin findings of these genetic conditions is important to aid in an early diagnosis, especially given that they all have the potential to involve internal organs such as the cardiovascular system and lungs.

More localized skin conditions are also represented here, including the serpiginous keratotic papules seen in elastosis perforans serpiginosa. This rare condition is more common in those with trisomy 21 (Down syndrome), but can also be seen in patients with some of the aforementioned connective tissue conditions such as EDS and Marfan syndrome.

Skin biopsy with subsequent staining for connective tissue fibers can be necessary and diagnostic for some of these conditions such as PXE. However, those patients with a suspected inherited condition with known gene mutation should be offered confirmatory genetic testing from the blood.

This portion of the atlas features these connective tissue diseases, among others, that affect the dermal fibrous and elastic tissues.

Fig. 25.1 Elastosis perforans serpiginosa.

Fig. 25.2 Elastosis perforans serpiginosa. *Courtesy Ken Greer, MD.*

Fig. 25.3 Elastosis perforans serpiginosa. *Courtesy Ken Greer, MD.*

Fig. 25.4 Elastosis perforans serpiginosa.

Fig. 25.5 Reactive perforating collagenosis. *Courtesy Steven Binnick, MD.*

Fig. 25.6 Reactive perforating collagenosis. *Courtesy Steven Binnick, MD.*

Fig. 25.7 Pseudoxanthoma elasticum.

Fig. 25.8 Pseudoxanthoma elasticum.

Fig. 25.9 Pseudoxanthoma elasticum.

Fig. 25.10 Pseudoxanthoma elasticum.

Fig. 25.11 Pseudoxanthoma elasticum.

Fig. 25.12 Pseudoxanthoma elasticum.

Fig. 25.13 Pseudoxanthoma elasticum.

Fig. 25.14 Pseudoxanthoma elasticum.

Fig. 25.15 Pseudoxanthoma elasticum.

Fig. 25.16 Pseudoxanthoma elasticum.

Fig. 25.17 Pseudoxanthoma elasticum–like papillary dermal elastolysis.

Fig. 25.18 Penicillamine elastopathy.

Fig. 25.19 Ehlers-Danlos syndrome.

Fig. 25.20 Ehlers-Danlos syndrome and elastosis perforans serpiginosa.

Fig. 25.21 Ehlers-Danlos syndrome.

Fig. 25.22 Ehlers-Danlos syndrome.

Fig. 25.23 Ehlers-Danlos syndrome.

Fig. 25.24 Ehlers-Danlos syndrome.

Fig. 25.25 Ehlers-Danlos syndrome. *Courtesy Steven Binnick, MD.*

Fig. 25.26 Ehlers-Danlos syndrome.

Fig. 25.27 Ehlers-Danlos syndrome.

Fig. 25.28 Ehlers-Danlos syndrome with scarring and molluscoid pseudotumor.

Fig. 25.29 Molluscoid pseudotumor.

Fig. 25.30 Ehlers-Danlos syndrome type IV with translucent skin.

Fig. 25.31 Ehlers Danlos syndrome with atrophic scar.

Fig. 25.32 Ehlers-Danlos syndrome.

Fig. 25.33 Shin of Ehlers-Danlos type VIII patient.

Fig. 25.34 Marfan syndrome.

Fig. 25.35 Cutis laxa.

Fig. 25.36 Cutis laxa.

Fig. 25.37 Neonatal cutis laxa.

Fig. 25.38 Blepharochalasis in Ascher syndrome. *Courtesy Ken Greer, MD.*

Fig. 25.39 Anetoderma.

Fig. 25.40 Anetoderma.

Fig. 25.41 Anetoderma of prematurity.

Fig. 25.42 Striae distensae.

Fig. 25.43 Striae distensae. *Courtesy Scott Norton, MD.*

Fig. 25.44 Striae distensae.

Fig. 25.45 Striae distensae.

Fig. 25.46 Elastotic striae.

Fig. 25.47 Elastotic striae.

Fig. 25.48 Osteogenesis imperfecta with blue sclera. *Courtesy Scott Norton, MD.*

Errors in Metabolism 26

This chapter provides images of a collection of conditions that result from errors in metabolism. Many of these diseases manifest in the skin secondary to the deposition of material such as amyloid, porphyrin, calcium, lipid, and urate crystals.

Amyloidosis includes systemic and localized cutaneous forms. Systemic amyloidosis is characterized clinically by scattered shiny, firm papules, plaques, and nodules; macroglossia; and, most commonly, easy bruising with the typical "pinched purpura." Cutaneous amyloidosis includes the keratinocyte-derived amyloid deposited in macular and lichenoid patterns, as well as the nodular, plasma cell-derived form.

Porphyrins are required to build heme, but when specific enzyme defects cause them to accumulate, they can cause tissue damage after being activated by visible light (400-410 nm). This interaction with light explains why porphyrias are conditions that demonstrate photosensitivity with vesicles, bullae, and erosions in the typical photodistributed pattern on the face, upper chest, and dorsal hands and forearms. Other clinical findings of note in porphyrias include hyperpigmentation, skin fragility, and hypertrichosis.

Calcinosis cutis has been categorized into dystrophic, metastatic, and iatrogenic, depending on the cause. All forms present with rock-hard papules, nodules, or plaques that can extrude whitish chalky material. Patient history, full physical examination, and laboratory investigations will help distinguish between these forms of calcinosis. Idiopathic calcinosis cutis also occurs in specific locations, such as the scrotum, where it often does not require further clinical workup.

Deposition of lipid in the skin leads to yellow- or orange-colored papules, plaques, or masses that are categorized clinically based on their anatomic location and morphology. These include tuberous and tendinous xanthomas that often occur over joints requiring differentiation from gout. Eruptive xanthomas present with widespread papules, whereas plane xanthomas are characterized by larger yellowish patches. Other more localized xanthomas include palmar xanthomas on the hands and xanthelasma palpebrarum on the eyelids. Although xanthelasmas can be found in the setting of normal lipid levels, all patients with xanthomas require a workup to confirm the diagnosis and screen for a wide range of hyperlipidemias.

This portion of the atlas includes the previously mentioned deposition-related conditions, the cutaneous manifestations of diabetes mellitus, and rarer syndromes, including lipoid proteinosis and Fabry disease (angiokeratoma corporis diffusum).

Fig. 26.1 Amyloidosis.

Fig. 26.2 Amyloidosis.

Fig. 26.3 Amyloidosis.

Fig. 26.4 Amyloidosis.

Fig. 26.5 Macroglossia in amyloidosis.

Fig. 26.6 Macroglossia in amyloidosis.

Fig. 26.7 Amyloidosis of the tongue.

Fig. 26.8 Amyloidosis.

Fig. 26.9 Amyloidosis.

Fig. 26.10 Amyloidosis.

Fig. 26.11 Amyloidosis.

Fig. 26.12 Amyloidosis with involvement of the nail matrix with resultant dystrophy. *Courtesy Robert Micheletti, MD.*

Fig. 26.13 Macular amyloidosis.

Fig. 26.14 Lichen amyloidosis.

Fig. 26.15 Lichen amyloidosis.

Fig. 26.16 Lichen amyloidosis.

Fig. 26.17 Lichen amyloidosis. *Courtesy Steven Binnick, MD.*

Fig. 26.18 Lichen amyloidosis.

Fig. 26.19 Lichen amyloidosis.

Fig. 26.20 Nodular amyloidosis.

Fig. 26.21 Nodular amyloidosis.

Fig. 26.22 Dyschromic amyloidosis. *Courtesy Vasanop Vachiramon, MD.*

Fig. 26.23 Porphyria cutanea tarda.

Fig. 26.24 Porphyria cutanea tarda.

Fig. 26.25 Porphyria cutanea tarda. *Courtesy Steven Binnick, MD.*

Fig. 26.26 Porphyria cutanea tarda in a patient with hepatoma.

Fig. 26.27 Porphyria cutanea tarda in a patient with hepatoma. *Courtesy Steven Binnick, MD.*

Fig. 26.28 Hypertrichosis in porphyria cutanea tarda.

Fig. 26.29 Pseudo–porphyria cutanea tarda. A 16-year-old girl who was taking tetracycline for acne.

Fig. 26.30 Sclerodemoid lesions in a patient with porphyria cutanea tarda.

Fig. 26.31 Erythropoietic protoporphyria in a neonate after bili-light exposure.

Fig. 26.32 Erythropoietic protoporphyria with scarring.

Fig. 26.33 Erythropoietic protoporphyria with scarring.

Fig. 26.34 Erythropoietic protoporphyria with scarring.

Fig. 26.35 Erythropoietic protoporphyria with scarring, thickening, and pebbling of the skin.

Fig. 26.36 Dystrophic calcinosis cutis.

Fig. 26.37 Calciphylaxis.

Fig. 26.38 Heel stick calcinosis.

Fig. 26.39 Scrotal calcinosis. *Courtesy Steven Binnick, MD.*

Fig. 26.40 Subepidermal calcified nodule.

Fig. 26.41 Calcinosis cutis.

Fig. 26.42 Tumoral calcinosis cutis.

Fig. 26.43 Osteoma cutis in acne scars.

Fig. 26.44 Osteoma cutis.

Fig. 26.45 Eruptive xanthomas.

Fig. 26.46 Eruptive xanthomas.

Fig. 26.47 Eruptive xanthomas.

Fig. 26.48 Type I hyperlipidemic eruptive xanthomas.

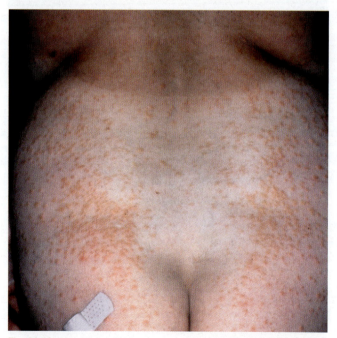

Fig. 26.49 Type I hyperlipidemic eruptive xanthomas.

Fig. 26.50 Tuberous xanthomas.

Fig. 26.51 Tuberous xanthomas.

Fig. 26.52 Tuberous xanthomas.

Fig. 26.53 Tuberous xanthoma.

Fig. 26.54 Tendinous xanthoma.

Fig. 26.55 Tendinous xanthomas.

Fig. 26.56 Homozygous hypercholesterolemia with intertriginous xanthomas.

Fig. 26.57 Homozygous hypercholesterolemia with intertriginous xanthomas.

Fig. 26.58 Xanthelasma.

Fig. 26.59 Xanthelasma.

Fig. 26.60 Plane xanthoma.

Fig. 26.61 Plane xanthoma.

Fig. 26.62 Primary biliary cirrhosis and tuberoeruptive xanthomas. *Courtesy Scott Norton, MD.*

Fig. 26.63 Palmar xanthomas in biliary cirrhosis.

Fig. 26.64 Palmar xanthomas in biliary cirrhosis. *Courtesy Steven Binnick, MD.*

Fig. 26.65 Plane xanthoma in biliary cirrhosis. *Courtesy Steven Binnick, MD.*

Fig. 26.66 Palmar xanthomas in Alagille syndrome. *Courtesy Steven Binnick, MD.*

Fig. 26.67 Cerebrotendinous xanthomas. *Courtesy Vikash Oza, MD.*

Fig. 26.68 Sitosterolemia.

Fig. 26.69 Tangier disease with residual yellow tonsils.

Fig. 26.70 Verruciform xanthoma.

Fig. 26.71 Verruciform xanthoma.

Fig. 26.72 Lipoid proteinosis.

Fig. 26.73 Lipoid proteinosis.

Fig. 26.74 Lipoid proteinosis.

Fig. 26.75 Lipoid proteinosis.

Fig. 26.76 Fabry disease. *Courtesy Ken Greer, MD.*

Fig. 26.77 Fabry disease.

Fig. 26.78 Necrobiosis lipoidica.

Fig. 26.79 Necrobiosis lipoidica.

Fig. 26.80 Necrobiosis lipoidica. *Courtesy Scott Norton, MD.*

Fig. 26.81 Necrobiosis lipoidica.

Fig. 26.82 Necrobiosis lipoidica.

Fig. 26.83 Diabetic dermopathy.

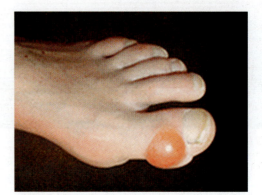

Fig. 26.84 Bullous diabetic dermatosis.

Fig. 26.85 Diabetic gangrene.

Fig. 26.86 Alkaptonuria.

Fig. 26.87 Alkaptonuria.

Fig. 26.88 Exogenous ochronosis.

Fig. 26.89 Exogenous ochronosis.

Fig. 26.90 Hunter syndrome. *Courtesy Paul Honig, MD.*

Fig. 26.91 Hunter syndrome.

Fig. 26.92 Gout.

Errors in metabolism

377

Fig. 26.93 Gout.

Fig. 26.94 Gout.

Fig. 26.95 Gout.

Fig. 26.96 Gout.

Fig. 26.97 Gout.

Genodermatoses and Congenital Anomalies 27

Genodermatoses include a variety of skin conditions due to underlying genetic mutations with and without associated systemic findings. New gene mutations are being discovered rapidly and allow for more definitive diagnoses in many of these conditions; however, recognizing the salient features on physical examination allows for more directed genetic testing.

Some genodermatoses will present at birth, such as epidermolysis bullosa with skin fragility or congenital ichthyoses with the presence of a collodion membrane. Other conditions manifest distinctive clinical findings in the neonatal period, as seen in the Blaschko linear vesicular and verrucous eruptions indicative of incontentia pigmenti. Childhood onset is more common for conditions like tuberous sclerosis (TS) or neurofibromatosis when patients begin to demonstrate more noticeable clinical stigmata such as angiofibromas or neurofibromas, respectively. Still other genodermatoses can present later during adolescence or early adulthood, including Darier disease with keratotic and crusted papules and plaques and Hailey-Hailey disease (familial benign chronic pemphigus) with reticulated, eroded flexural plaques.

Photosensitivity can be seen in several genodermatoses, including the telangiectatic patches of Bloom syndrome; the poikiloderma of Rothmund-Thomson syndrome; and the lentigines, sun damage, and early skin cancers seen in xeroderma pigmentosa.

A thorough evaluation of these conditions should include examination of the hair, nails, mucosa, and teeth. Screening for associated symptoms is important, such as lack of sweating present in several forms of ectodermal dysplasia or developmental delays and seizures that can be present in several genodermatoses such as epidermal nevus syndrome or TS. Finally, family history can be useful in determining the inheritance pattern and to narrow genetic testing.

This portion of the atlas includes a wide variety of genodermatoses and congenital anomalies to aid the clinician in identifying the clinical clues that help differentiate these diseases and often guide genetic testing when appropriate.

Fig. 27.1 Incontinentia pigmenti, early inflammatory phase.

Fig. 27.2 Incontinentia pigmenti with verrucous lesions. *Courtesy Paul Honig, MD.*

Fig. 27.3 Incontinentia pigmenti with verrucous lesions.

Fig. 27.4 Incontinentia pigmenti with pigmentary lesions. *Courtesy Paul Honig, MD.*

Fig. 27.5 Incontinentia pigmenti with pigmentary lesions.

Fig. 27.6 Pigmentary mosaicism (previously Hypomelanosis of Ito). *Courtesy Department of Dermatology, Keio University School of Medicine, Tokyo, Japan.*

Fig. 27.7 Conradi-Hunermann syndrome.

Fig. 27.8 Conradi-Hunermann syndrome.

Fig. 27.9 Turner syndrome with congenital lymphedema. *Courtesy Steven Binnick, MD.*

Fig. 27.10 Noonan syndrome.

Fig. 27.11 Noonan syndrome with lymphedema and chylous discharge.

Fig. 27.12 Noonan syndrome with multiple lentigines (previously LEOPARD syndrome). *Courtesy Paul Honig, MD.*

Fig. 27.13 Tuberous sclerosis with angiofibromas and gingivival hypertrophy from taking phenytoin for his TS-related seizure disorder. *Courtesy Scott Norton, MD.*

Fig. 27.14 Tuberous sclerosis with angiofibromas.

Fig. 27.15 Tuberous sclerosis with periungual fibromas.

Fig. 27.16 Tuberous sclerosis with ash leaf macule.

Fig. 27.17 Tuberous sclerosis with ash leaf macule. *Courtesy Steven Binnick, MD.*

Fig. 27.18 Tuberous sclerosis with paintbrush-type white streaks.

Fig. 27.19 Tuberous sclerosis with shagreen plaque.

Fig. 27.20 Tuberous sclerosis with fibrous forehead plaque.

Fig. 27.21 Tuberous sclerosis with dental enamel pit.

Fig. 27.22 Neurofibromatosis.

Fig. 27.23 Neurofibromatosis. *Courtesy Steven Binnick, MD.*

Fig. 27.24 Neurofibromatosis.

Fig. 27.25 Neurofibromatosis. *Courtesy Steven Binnick, MD.*

Fig. 27.26 Neurofibromatosis; the areola are characteristically involved.

Fig. 27.27 Neurofibromatosis with café-au-lait macule.

Fig. 27.28 Neurofibromatosis with axillary freckling.

Fig. 27.29 Neurofibromatosis with plexiform neurofibroma.

Fig. 27.30 Neurofibromatosis with plexiform neurofibroma.

Fig. 27.31 Neurofibromatosis with a malignant peripheral nerve sheath tumor.

Fig. 27.32 Segmental neurofibromatosis.

Fig. 27.33 Proteus syndrome with connective tissue nevus.

Fig. 27.34 Proteus syndrome with connective tissue nevus.

Fig. 27.35 Proteus syndrome with epidermal nevus.

Fig. 27.36 Proteus syndrome. *Courtesy Curt Samlaska, MD.*

Fig. 27.37 Ataxia telangiectasia.

Fig. 27.38 Epidermolysis bullosa simplex, generalized.

Fig. 27.39 Epidermolysis bullosa simplex, generalized. *Courtesy Scott Norton, MD.*

Fig. 27.40 Epidermolysis bullosa simplex, localized.

Fig. 27.41 Junctional epidermolysis bullosa.

Fig. 27.42 Junctional epidermolysis bullosa.

Fig. 27.43 Bart syndrome.

Fig. 27.44 Dominant dystrophic epidermolysis bullosa.

Fig. 27.45 Dominant dystrophic epidermolysis bullosa.

Fig. 27.46 Recessive dystrophic epidermolysis bullosa.

Fig. 27.47 Recessive dystrophic epidermolysis bullosa.

Fig. 27.48 Hailey-Hailey disease. *Courtesy Steven Binnick, MD.*

Fig. 27.49 Hailey–Hailey disease.

Fig. 27.50 Hailey–Hailey disease.

Fig. 27.51 Hailey–Hailey disease.

Fig. 27.52 Ichthyosis vulgaris.

Fig. 27.53 Ichthyosis vulgaris. *Courtesy Steven Binnick, MD.*

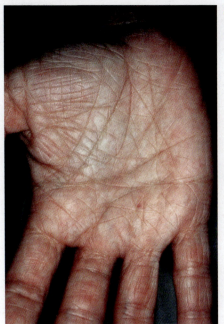

Fig. 27.54 Ichthyosis vulgaris with hyperlinear palms.

Fig. 27.55 X-linked ichthyosis.

Fig. 27.56 X-linked ichthyosis.

Fig. 27.57 X-linked ichthyosis.

Fig. 27.58 Autosomal-recessive congenital ichthyosis with collodion membrane.

Fig. 27.59 Autosomal-recessive congenital ichthyosis with collodion membrane due to transglutaminase gene mutation.

Fig. 27.60 Autosomal-recessive congenital ichthyosis lamellar phenotype due to transglutaminase gene mutation.

Fig. 27.61 Congenital ichthyosiform erythroderma. *Courtesy Scott Norton, MD.*

Fig. 27.62 Congenital ichthyosiform erythroderma. *Courtesy Scott Norton, MD.*

Fig. 27.63 Harlequin fetus. *Courtesy Scott Norton, MD.*

Fig. 27.64 Epidermolytic ichthyosis.

Fig. 27.65 Epidermolytic ichthyosis.

Fig. 27.66 Epidermolytic ichthyosis.

Fig. 27.67 Netherton syndrome. *Courtesy Scott Norton, MD.*

Fig. 27.68 Netherton syndrome. *Courtesy Scott Norton, MD.*

Fig. 27.69 Netherton syndrome.

Fig. 27.70 Netherton syndrome.

Fig. 27.71 Netherton syndrome.

Fig. 27.72 Keratitis ichthyosis deafness syndrome. *Courtesy Paul Honig, MD.*

Fig. 27.73 Keratitis ichthyosis deafness syndrome.

Fig. 27.74 Sjögren-Larsson syndrome.

Fig. 27.75 Congenital hemidysplasia with ichthyosiform erythroderma and limb defects (child) syndrome. *Courtesy Paul Honig, MD.*

Fig. 27.76 Erythrokeratoderma variabilis. *Courtesy Ken Greer, MD.*

Fig. 27.77 Progressive symmetric erythrokeratoderma. *Courtesy Ken Greer, MD.*

Fig. 27-78 Porokeratosis.

Fig. 27.79 Porokeratosis.

Fig. 27.80 Disseminated superficial actinic porokeratosis.

Fig. 27.81 Porokeratotic eccrine and osteal duct nevus.

Fig. 27.82 Darier disease.

Fig. 27.83 Darier disease.

Fig. 27.84 Darier disease.

Fig. 27.85 Darier disease.

Fig. 27.86 Darier disease. *Courtesy Curt Samlaska, MD.*

Fig. 27.87 Darier disease.

Fig. 27.88 Darier disease.

Fig. 27.89 Darier disease.

Fig. 27.90 Darier disease.

Fig. 27.91 Darier disease.

Fig. 27.92 Acrokeratosis verruciformis of Hopf.

Fig. 27.93 Pachyonychia congenita.

Fig. 27.94 Pachyonychia congenita.

Fig. 27.95 Pachyonychia congenita.

Fig. 27.96 Pachyonychia congenita.

Fig. 27.97 Pachyonychia congenita.

Fig. 27.98 Dyskeratosis congenita.

Fig. 27.99 Dyskeratosis congenita.

Fig. 27.100 Dyskeratosis congenita.

Fig. 27.101 Dyskeratosis congenita.

Fig. 27.102 Hypohidrotic X-linked ectodermal dysplasia. *Courtesy Scott Bartlett, MD.*

Fig. 27.103 Hypohidrotic X-linked ectodermal dysplasia.

Fig. 27.104 Hypohidrotic X-linked ectodermal dysplasia.

Fig. 27.105 Hypohidrotic X-linked ectodermal dysplasia.

Fig. 27.106 Hidrotic ectodermal dysplasia.

Fig. 27.107 Hidrotic ectodermal dysplasia.

Fig. 27.108 Ankyloblepharon-ectodermal dysplasia-clefting

Fig. 27.109 Ectrodactyly ectodermal dysplasia-clefting.

Fig. 27.110 Ectrodactyly ectodermal dysplasia-clefting.

Fig. 27.111 Cutis verticis gyrata.

Fig. 27.112 Cutis verticis gyrata. *Courtesy Steven Binnick, MD.*

Fig. 27.113 Aplasia cutis congenita.

Fig. 27.114 Hair collar sign.

Fig. 27.115 Goltz syndrome. *Courtesy Paul Honig, MD.*

Fig. 27.116 Goltz syndrome.

Fig. 27.117 Goltz syndrome.

Fig. 27.118 Werner syndrome.

Fig. 27.119 Werner syndrome.

Fig. 27.120 Werner syndrome.

Fig. 27.121 Werner syndrome.

Fig. 27.122 Progeria.

Fig. 27.123 Xeroderma pigmentosum. *Courtesy Kenneth Kraemer, MD. First published in Bradford PT, Goldstein AM, Tamura D, et al: Cancer and neurologic degeneration in xeroderma pigmentosum. J Med Genet 2011; 48: 168–176.*

Fig. 27.124 Xeroderma pigmentosum. *Courtesy Kenneth Kraemer, MD. First published in Bradford PT, Goldstein AM, Tamura D, et al: Cancer and neurologic degeneration in xeroderma pigmentosum. J Med Genet 2011; 48: 168–176.*

Fig. 27.125 Xeroderma pigmentosum. *Courtesy Kenneth Kraemer, MD. First published in Bradford PT, Goldstein AM, Tamura D, et al: Cancer and neurologic degeneration in xeroderma pigmentosum. J Med Genet 2011; 48: 168–176.*

Fig. 27.126 Xeroderma pigmentosum. *Courtesy Kenneth Kraemer, MD. First published in Mahindra P, DiGiovanna JJ, Tamura D, et al: Skin cancers, blindness and anterior tongue mass in African brothers. J. Amer Acad Dermatol 2008; 59: 881–886.*

Fig. 27.127 Cockayne syndrome. *Courtesy Kenneth Kraemer, MD. First published in Lindenbaum,Y., Dickson, D.W., Rosenbaum, P., Kraemer, K.H., et al.: Xeroderma pigmentosum/Cockayne Syndrome (XP/CS) complex. Eur J Child Neurol 2001; 5: 225–242.*

Fig. 27.128 Cockayne-xeroderma pigmentosum syndrome complex. *Courtesy Kenneth Kraemer, MD. First published in Lindenbaum,Y., Dickson, D.W., Rosenbaum, P., Kraemer, K.H., et al.: Xeroderma pigmentosum/Cockayne Syndrome (XP/CS) complex. Eur J Child Neurol 2001; 5: 225–242.*

Fig. 27.129 Trichothiodystrophy. *Courtesy Kenneth Kraemer, MD. First published in Liang, C., Kraemer, K.H., Morris, A., et al: Characterization of tiger tail banding and hair shaft abnormalities in trichothiodystrophy J. American Acad. Dermatol. 2005; 52: 224–232.*

Fig. 27.130 Bloom syndrome.

Fig. 27.131 Rothmund-Thomson syndrome.

Fig. 27.132 Rothmund-Thomson syndrome.

Fig. 27.133 Rothmund-Thomson syndrome.

Fig. 27.134 Apert syndrome.

Fig. 27.135 Apert syndrome.

Fig. 27.136 Trichorhinophalangeal syndrome.

Fig. 27.137 Trichorhinophalangeal syndrome.

Fig. 27.138 Keratosis pilaris.

Fig. 27.139 Ulerythema ophrogenes.

Fig. 27.140 Keratosis follicularis spinulosa decalvans.

Dermal and Subcutaneous Tumors 28

Vascular tumors range from red to blue, depending on the degree of vascular stasis and deoxygenation of hemoglobin. When associated with thrombosis or consumptive coagulopathy, the lesions often become hard and tender. The clinician should attempt to distinguish vascular proliferative lesions from vascular malformations, as the former tend to respond to beta blockers, whereas the latter do not. Malformations include nevus flammeus, salmon patch, nevus anemicus, and cutis marmorata telangiectatica congenita. Some vascular malformations are associated with overgrowth of surrounding tissues and can lead to considerable morbidity. This portion of the atlas will focus on the clinical findings of dermal tumors, including fibrous and vascular proliferations, as well as growths, in addition to those composed of muscles, nerves, and fatty tissue.

A biopsy may be required for the definitive diagnosis of dermal neoplasms, but the color, morphology, and distribution of the lesions can often lead to an accurate clinical diagnosis. Dermatofibromas present as firm, pink-to brown dermal nodules with overlying epidermal acanthosis imparting a dull or velvety appearance to the skin. A characteristic dimpling sign occurs when the surrounding skin is compressed laterally. Granular cell tumors tend to be larger, but are accompanied by a similar velvety or verrucous appearance of the overlying skin. In contrast, dermatofibrosarcoma protuberans presents with a multinodular appearance with overlying epidermal atrophy imparting a taught, glossy appearance to the skin. All of these tumors are quite firm to palpation in contrast to the soft rubbery or gelatinous feel of a neurofibroma.

Fig. 28.1 Phacomatosis pigmentovascularis. *Courtesy Department of Dermatology, Keio University School of Medicine, Tokyo, Japan.*

Fig. 28.2 Phacomatosis pigmentovascularis.

Fig. 28.3 PIK3CA-related segmental overgrowth syndrome.

Fig. 28.4 PIK3CA-related segmental overgrowth syndrome.

Fig. 28.5 Nevus anemicus.

Fig. 28.6 Nevus anemicus.

Fig. 28.7 Cutis marmorata telangiectatica congenita. *Courtesy Paul Honig, MD.*

Fig. 28.8 Nevus simplex. *Courtesy Steven Binnick, MD.*

Fig. 28.9 Nevus simplex.

Fig. 28.10 Nevus simplex.

Fig. 28.11 Capillary malformation (port-wine stain) with Sturge-Weber syndrome.

Fig. 28.12 Capillary malformation (port-wine stain) with Sturge-Weber syndrome.

Fig. 28.13 Capillary malformation (port-wine stain).

Fig. 28.14 Capillary malformation (port-wine stain).

Fig. 28.15 RASA1-associated capillary malformation-arteriovenous malformation syndrome.

Fig. 28.16 Cavernous venous malformation.

Fig. 28.17 Cavernous venous malformation.

Fig. 28.18 Cavernous venous malformation.

Fig. 28.19 Venous malformation.

Fig. 28.20 Blue rubber bleb syndrome.

Fig. 28.21 Maffucci syndrome.

Fig. 28.22 Klippel-Trenaunay syndrome.

Fig. 28.23 Arteriovenous fistula.

Fig. 28.24 Microcystic lymphatic malformation.

Fig. 28.25 Oral lymphatic malformation.

Fig. 28.26 Superficial lymphatic malformation.

Fig. 28.27 Venolymphatic malformation. *Courtesy Ken Greer, MD.*

Fig. 28.28 Acquired lymphangiectasia after surgery and radiation therapy for breast cancer. Redness is irritation from chylous discharge.

Fig. 28.29 Deep lymphatic malformation.

Fig. 28.30 Spider angioma. *Courtesy Steven Binnick, MD.*

Fig. 28.31 Venous lakes. *Courtesy Ken Greer, MD.*

Fig. 28.32 Generalized essential telangiectasia. *Courtesy Steven Binnick, MD.*

Fig. 28.33 Unilateral nevoid telangiectasia.

Fig. 28.34 Angiokeratoma circumscriptum. *Courtesy Steven Binnick, MD.*

Fig. 28.35 Angiokeratoma circumscriptum. *Courtesy Steven Binnick, MD.*

Fig. 28.36 Angiokeratoma of Mibelli.

Fig. 28.37 Angiokeratoma of Fordyce.

Fig. 28.38 Angiokeratoma of Fordyce.

Fig. 28.39 Angiokeratoma of Fordyce.

Fig. 28.40 Angiokeratoma of Fordyce.

Fig. 28.41 Angiokeratoma of Fordyce.

Fig. 28.42 Angiolymphoid hyperplasia with eosinophilia.

Fig. 28.43 Pyogenic granuloma. *Courtesy Steven Binnick, MD.*

Fig. 28.44 Pyogenic granuloma. *Courtesy Steven Binnick, MD.*

Fig. 28.45 Pyogenic granuloma. *Courtesy Steven Binnick, MD.*

Fig. 28.46 Pyogenic granuloma. *Courtesy Steven Binnick, MD.*

Fig. 28.47 Recurrent pyogenic granulomas with satellite lesions.

Fig. 28.48 Angioma serpiginosum.

Fig. 28.49 Infantile hemangioma. *Courtesy Steven Binnick, MD.*

Fig. 28.50 Infantile hemangioma.

Fig. 28.51 Infantile hemangioma with ulceration.

Fig. 28.52 Infantile hemangioma with ulceration.

Fig. 28.53 Involuting infantile hemangioma.

Fig. 28.54 Involuting infantile hemangioma.

Fig. 28.55 PHACE syndrome.

Fig. 28.56 LUMBAR syndrome. *Courtesy Scott Norton, MD.*

Fig. 28.57 Diffuse neonatal hemangiomatosis.

Fig. 28.58 Cherry angiomas and costal fringe telangiectases.

Fig. 28.59 Targetoid hemosiderotic hemangioma.

Fig. 28.60 Tufted angioma.

Fig. 28.61 Kaposiform hemangioendothelioma.

Fig. 28.62 Kasabach-Merritt syndrome.

Fig. 28.63 Glomangioma.

Fig. 28.64 Glomangioma.

Fig. 28.65 Diffuse dermal angiomatosis.

Fig. 28.66 Spindle cell hemangioma.

Fig. 28.67 Kaposi sarcoma in an HIV-infected patient.

Fig. 28.68 Kaposi sarcoma in an HIV-infected patient; the palate is commonly involved.

Fig. 28.69 Kaposi sarcoma in an HIV-infected patient; the linear elongated lesions along skin lines are characteristic.

Fig. 28.70 Kaposi sarcoma in an HIV-infected patient. *Courtesy Steven Binnick, MD.*

Fig. 28.71 Angiosarcoma. *Courtesy Steven Binnick, MD.*

Fig. 28.72 Angiosarcoma.

Fig. 28.73 Keloid. *Courtesy Steven Binnick, MD.*

Fig. 28.74 Keloid. *Courtesy Steven Binnick, MD.*

Fig. 28.75 Keloid. *Courtesy Steven Binnick, MD.*

Fig. 28.76 Ulcerated keloids.

Fig. 28.77 Dupuytren contracture.

Fig. 28.78 Plantar fibromatosis.

Fig. 28.79 Knuckle pads. *Courtesy Curt Samlaska, MD.*

Fig. 28.80 Pachydermodactyly.

Fig. 28.81 Solitary congenital myofibroma.

Fig. 28.82 Infantile digital fibromas.

Fig. 28.83 Infantile digital fibromas. *Courtesy Sheilagh Maguiness, MD.*

Fig. 28.84 Giant cell tumor of the tendon sheath.

Fig. 28.85 Ainhum.

Fig. 28.86 Connective tissue nevus.

Fig. 28.87 Connective tissue nevus.

Fig. 28.88 Buschke-Ollendorff syndrome.

Fig. 28.89 Fibrous papule of the nose. *Courtesy Curt Samlaska, MD.*

Fig. 28.90 Pearly penile papules.

Fig. 28.91 Acquired digital fibrokeratoma. *Courtesy Debabrata Bandyopadhyay.*

Fig. 28.92 Acquired digital fibrokeratoma.

Fig. 28.93 Subungual exostosis. *Courtesy Curt Samlaska, MD.*

Fig. 28.94 Chondrodermatitis nodularis chronica helices.

Fig. 28.95 Skin tag. *Courtesy Steven Binnick, MD.*

Fig. 28.96 Skin tags. *Courtesy Steven Binnick, MD.*

Fig. 28.97 Dermatofibroma. *Courtesy Steven Binnick, MD.*

Fig. 28.98 Dermatofibroma. *Courtesy Steven Binnick, MD.*

Fig. 28.99 Dermatofibroma.

Fig. 28.100 Multiple dermatofibromas. *Courtesy Ken Greer, MD.*

Fig. 28.101 Dermal dendrocyte hamartoma.

Fig. 28.102 Dermatofibroma sarcoma protuberans. *Courtesy Ken Greer, MD.*

Fig. 28.103 Dermatofibroma sarcoma protuberans. *Courtesy Chris Miller, MD.*

Fig. 28.104 Atypical fibroxanthoma. *Courtesy Chris Miller, MD.*

Fig. 28.105 Atypical fibroxanthoma.

Fig. 28.106 Epithelioid sarcoma.

Fig. 28.107 Solitary mastocytoma.

Fig. 28.108 Darier sign mastocytoma. *Courtesy Steven Binnick, MD.*

Fig. 28.109 Darier sign mastocytoma. *Courtesy Steven Binnick, MD.*

Fig. 28.110 Bullous mastocytosis. *Courtesy Steven Binnick, MD.*

Fig. 28.111 Urticaria pigmentosa.

Fig. 28.112 Mastocytosis.

Fig. 28.113 Mastocytosis.

Fig. 28.114 Mastocytosis.

Fig. 28.115 Generalized adult mastocytosis.

Fig. 28.116 Generalized adult mastocytosis.

Fig. 28.117 Solitary neurofibroma. *Courtesy Steven Binnick, MD.*

Fig. 28.118 Granular cell tumor.

Fig. 28.119 Granular cell tumor.

Fig. 28.120 Multiple granular cell tumor.

Fig. 28.121 Neuroma.

Fig. 28.122 Multiple mucosal neuroma syndrome.

Fig. 28.123 Neurilemmoma.

Fig. 28.124 Nasal glioma. *Courtesy Scott Bartlett, MD.*

Fig. 28.125 Encephalocele. *Courtesy Scott Bartlett, MD.*

Fig. 28.126 Encephalocele.

Fig. 28.127 Encephalocele. *Courtesy Paul Honig, MD.*

Fig. 28.128 Lipoma. *Courtesy Steven Binnick, MD.*

Fig. 28.129 Multiple lipomas.

Fig. 28.130 Multiple lipomas.

Fig. 28.131 Multiple lipomas.

Fig. 28.132 Nevus lipomatosis superficialis.

Fig. 28.133 Michelin tire baby.

Fig. 28.134 Leiomyoma. *Courtesy Steven Binnick, MD.*

Fig. 28.135 Multiple leiomyomas.

Fig. 28.136 Multiple leiomyomas. *Courtesy Steven Binnick, MD.*

Fig. 28.137 Multiple leiomyomas. *Courtesy Debabrata Bandyopadhyay.*

Fig. 28.138 Multiple leiomyomas.

Fig. 28.139 Smooth muscle hamartoma.

Fig. 28.140 Leiomyosarcoma.

Fig. 28.141 Leiomyosarcoma. *Courtesy Chris Miller, MD.*

Fig. 28.142 Cutaneous endometriosis. *Courtesy Scott Norton, MD.*

Fig. 28.143 Teratoma.

Fig. 28.144 Ductal breast cancer. *Courtesy Steven Binnick, MD.*

Fig. 28.145 Inflammatory breast cancer.

Fig. 28.146 Carcinoma erysipeloides.

Fig. 28.147 Alopecia neoplastica (breast cancer).

Fig. 28.148 Male breast cancer metastases.

Fig. 28.149 Lung cancer metastases.

Fig. 28.150 Lung cancer metastases.

Fig. 28.151 Lung cancer metastases.

Fig. 28.152 Prostate cancer metastases.

Fig. 28.153 Prostate cancer metastases.

Fig. 28.154 Uterine cancer metastases (Sister Mary Joseph nodule).

Fig. 28.155 Glucagonoma.

Fig. 28.156 Glucagonoma.

Fig. 28.157 Glucagonoma.

Fig. 28.158 Bazex syndrome.

Fig. 28.159 Paraneoplastic pemphigus. *Courtesy Department of Dermatology, Keio University School of Medicine, Tokyo, Japan.*

Fig. 28.160 Hypertrophic osteoarthropathy from lung cancer.

Fig. 28.161 Acquired ichthyosis in a myeloma patient.

Fig. 28.162 Pachydermoperiostosis secondary to cancer.

Fig. 28.163 Carcinoid syndrome.

Epidermal Nevi, Neoplasms, and Cysts — 29

Epidermal neoplasms commonly present with hyperkeratosis, acanthosis, or papillomatosis. These may manifest clinically as a cutaneous horn, scale, palpable induration, a velvety or filiform appearance, or a smooth lesion raised above the surrounding skin surface. As an example, epidermal nevi tend to be raised and linear in configuration, following Blaschko lines. They may be hyperpigmented, hypopigmented, fleshy, or keratotic in appearance.

Cysts and dermal epithelial neoplasms displace the overlying skin and may produce overlying atrophy, erythema, or telangiectasia. The presence of tumor-associated vascularity lends a red or blue appearance, depending on the speed of blood flow and oxygen saturation of the blood. The presence of cytoplasm lends a yellow appearance due to carotenoids dissolved in the aqueous phase of cytoplasm. A brown appearance most commonly relates to melanin within the epithelial cells and underlying dermis, but can also be a result of dermal hemosiderin or lipofuscin deposition. Lipofuscin dissolved in apocrine sweat often lends a blue appearance to portions of sweat gland tumors as a result of diffraction of light (the Tyndall effect). Sebaceous elements lend a yellow or orange appearance. An appreciation of the color, morphology, and distribution of the lesions will help the physician narrow the differential diagnosis.

Fig. 29.2 Epidermal nevus.

Fig. 29.1 Epidermal nevus.

Fig. 29.3 Epidermal nevus.

Fig. 29.4 CLOVE syndrome.

Fig. 29.5 Nevus comedonicus.

Fig. 29.6 Schimmelpenning syndrome with a lipodermoid of the conjunctiva.

Fig. 29.7 Inflammatory linear verrucous epidermal nevus.

Fig. 29.8 Clear cell acanthoma. *Courtesy Ken Greer, MD.*

Fig. 29.9 Multiple clear cell acanthomas.

Fig. 29.10 Warty dyskeratomas.

Fig. 29.11 Seborrheic keratosis. *Courtesy Steven Binnick, MD.*

Fig. 29.12 Seborrheic keratosis. *Courtesy Steven Binnick, MD.*

Fig. 29.13 Seborrheic keratosis. *Courtesy Steven Binnick, MD.*

Fig. 29.14 Seborrheic keratosis.

Fig. 29.15 Seborrheic keratosis.

Fig. 29.16 Dermatosis papulosa nigra. *Courtesy Steven Binnick, MD.*

Fig. 29.17 Dermatosis papulosa nigra.

Fig. 29.18 Stucco keratosis.

Fig. 29.19 Flegel disease.

Fig. 29.20 Benign lichenoid keratoses.

Fig. 29.21 Arsenical keratoses.

Fig. 29.22 Actinic keratoses.

Fig. 29.23 Actinic keratoses.

Fig. 29.24 Actinic keratoses in vitiliginous skin.

Fig. 29.25 Hypertrophic actinic keratosis.

Fig. 29.26 Cutaneous horn. *Courtesy Steven Binnick, MD.*

Fig. 29.27 Cutaneous horn. *Courtesy Debabrata Bandyopadhyay.*

Fig. 29.28 Keratoacanthoma. *Courtesy Curt Samlaska, MD.*

Fig. 29.29 Keratoacanthoma. *Courtesy Steven Binnick, MD.*

Fig. 29.30 Keratoacanthoma.

Fig. 29.31 Multiple keratoacanthomas.

Fig. 29.32 Eruptive keratoacanthoma.

Fig. 29.33 Eruptive keratoacanthoma.

Fig. 29.34 Basal cell carcinoma.

Fig. 29.35 Basal cell carcinoma.

Fig. 29.36 Basal cell carcinoma.

Fig. 29.37 Basal cell carcinoma.

Fig. 29.38 Basal cell carcinoma. *Courtesy Steven Binnick, MD.*

Fig. 29.39 Superficial basal cell carcinoma.

Fig. 29.40 Pigmented basal cell carcinoma. *Courtesy Curt Samlaska, MD.*

Fig. 29.41 Pigmented basal cell carcinoma. *Courtesy Debabrata Bandyopadhyay, MD.*

Fig. 29.42 Morpheaform basal cell carcinoma. *Courtesy Steven Binnick, MD.*

Fig. 29.43 Basal cell carcinoma.

Fig. 29.44 Large basal cell carcinoma.

Fig. 29.45 Aggressive basal cell carcinoma.

Fig. 29.46 Multiple basal cell carcinomas in a radiation site. *Courtesy Steven Binnick, MD.*

Fig. 29.47 Basal cell nevus syndrome with skin tag–like basal cell carcinomas. *Courtesy Ken Greer, MD.*

Fig. 29.48 Basal cell nevus syndrome. *Courtesy Steven Binnick, MD.*

Fig. 29.49 Basal cell nevus syndrome. *Courtesy Steven Binnick, MD.*

Fig. 29.50 Basal cell nevus syndrome. *Courtesy Steven Binnick, MD.*

Fig. 29.51 Palmar pits in basal cell nevus syndrome.

Fig. 29.52 Squamous cell carcinoma.

Fig. 29.53 Squamous cell carcinoma.

Fig. 29.54 Squamous cell carcinoma.

Fig. 29.55 Squamous cell carcinoma.

Fig. 29.56 Squamous cell carcinoma. *Courtesy Shyam Verma, MBBS, DVD.*

Fig. 29.57 Squamous cell carcinoma in an African American patient. *Courtesy Steven Binnick, MD.*

Fig. 29.58 Squamous cell carcinoma in a burn scar. *Courtesy Steven Binnick, MD.*

Fig. 29.59 Verrucous carcinoma.

Fig. 29.60 Bowen disease.

Fig. 29.61 Bowen disease. *Courtesy Steven Binnick, MD.*

Fig. 29.62 Bowen disease.

Fig. 29.63 Bowen disease with squamous cell carcinoma.

Fig. 29.64 Bowen disease.

Fig. 29.65 Pigmented multicentric Bowen disease.

Fig. 29.66 Erythroplasia of Queyrat.

Fig. 29.67 Zoon balanitis.

Fig. 29.68 Paget disease of the breast. *Courtesy Steven Binnick, MD.*

Fig. 29.69 Paget disease of the breast. *Courtesy Steven Binnick, MD.*

Fig. 29.70 Extramammary Paget disease. *Courtesy Steven Binnick, MD.*

Fig. 29.71 Extramammary Paget disease. *Courtesy Steven Binnick, MD.*

Fig. 29.72 Merkel cell carcinoma. *Courtesy Thuzar Shin, MD, PhD.*

Fig. 29.73 Merkel cell carcinoma. *Courtesy Chris Miller, MD.*

Fig. 29.74 Nevus sebaceous. *Courtesy Steven Binnick, MD.*

Fig. 29.75 Nevus sebaceous.

Fig. 29.76 Nevus sebaceous with basal cell carcinoma. *Courtesy Steven Binnick, MD.*

Fig. 29.77 Sebaceous hyperplasia. *Courtesy Steven Binnick, MD.*

Fig. 29.78 Sebaceous adenomas of Muir Torre syndrome. *Courtesy Steven Binnick, MD.*

Fig. 29.79 Sebaceous adenomas of Muir Torre syndrome.

Fig. 29.80 Sebaceous carcinoma.

Fig. 29.81 Syringomas. *Courtesy Steven Binnick, MD.*

Fig. 29.82 Syringomas. *Courtesy Steven Binnick, MD.*

Fig. 29.83 Syringomas. *Courtesy Steven Binnick, MD.*

Fig. 29.84 Syringomas.

Fig. 29.85 Syringomas.

Fig. 29.86 Syringomas.

Fig. 29.87 Syringomas.

Fig. 29.88 Hidrocystoma.

Fig. 29.89 Hidrocystoma.

Fig. 29.90 Hidrocystoma. *Courtesy Steven Binnick, MD.*

Fig. 29.91 Multiple hidrocystomas.

Fig. 29.92 Eccrine poroma.

Fig. 29.93 Eccrine poroma.

Fig. 29.94 Nodular hidradenoma. *Courtesy Steven Binnick, MD.*

Fig. 29.95 Eccrine acrospiroma.

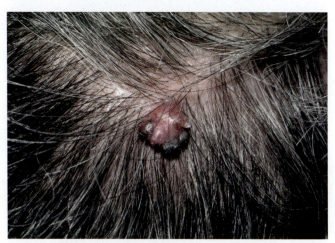

Fig. 29.96 Eccrine spiradenoma. *Courtesy Steven Binnick, MD.*

Fig. 29.97 Multiple acrospiromas. *Courtesy Steven Binnick, MD.*

Fig. 29.98 Dermal duct tumor. *Courtesy Steven Binnick, MD.*

Fig. 29.99 Eccrine porocarcinoma.

Fig. 29.100 Eccrine porocarcinoma. *Courtesy Chris Miller, MD.*

Fig. 29.101 Cylindroma.

Fig. 29.102 Multiple cylindromas.

Fig. 29.103 Chondroid syringoma.

Fig. 29.104 Syringocystadenoma papilliferum.

Fig. 29.105 Syringocystadenoma papilliferum.

Fig. 29.106 Syringocystadenoma papilliferum in nevus sebaceous. *Courtesy Steven Binnick, MD.*

Fig. 29.107 Microcystic adnexal carcinoma. *Courtesy Chris Miller, MD.*

Fig. 29.108 Eccrine carcinoma.

Fig. 29.109 Pilomatricoma. *Courtesy Scott Bartlett, MD.*

Fig. 29.110 Pilomatricoma.

Fig. 29.111 Pilomatricoma. *Courtesy Curt Samlaska, MD.*

Fig. 29.112 Trichofolliculoma.

Fig. 29.113 Brooke-Spiegler syndrome.

Fig. 29.114 Brooke-Spiegler syndrome.

Fig. 29.115 Solitary trichoepithelioma.

Fig. 29.116 Giant trichoepithelioma. *Courtesy Patrick Carrington, MD.*

Fig. 29.117 Desmoplastic trichoepithelioma.

Fig. 29.118 Solitary trichilemmoma.

Fig. 29.119 Cowden syndrome.

Fig. 29.120 Cowden syndrome.

Fig. 29.121 Oral papillomas in Cowden syndrome.

Fig. 29.122 Sclerotic fibroma.

Fig. 29.123 Birt-Hogg-Dubé syndrome.

Fig. 29.124 Birt-Hogg-Dubé syndrome.

Fig. 29.125 Birt-Hogg-Dubé syndrome.

Fig. 29.126 Birt-Hogg-Dubé syndrome.

Fig. 29.127 Pore of Winer.

Fig. 29.128 Basaloid follicular hamartoma.

Fig. 29.129 Tumor of the follicular infundibulum.

Fig. 29.130 Epidermal inclusion cyst.

Fig. 29.131 Inflamed epidermal inclusion cyst. *Courtesy Steven Binnick, MD.*

Fig. 29.132 Scrotal cysts.

Fig. 29.133 Labial cysts. *Courtesy Steven Binnick, MD.*

Fig. 29.134 Pilar cyst.

Fig. 29.135 Proliferating pilar cyst.

Fig. 29.136 Dermoid cyst. *Courtesy Scott Bartlett, MD.*

Fig. 29.137 Dermoid cyst. *Courtesy Scott Norton, MD.*

Fig. 29.138 Pilonidal cyst. *Courtesy Scott Norton, MD.*

Fig. 29.139 Steatocystoma multiplex. *Courtesy Steven Binnick, MD.*

Fig. 29.140 Steatocystoma multiplex.

Fig. 29.141 Steatocystoma multiplex. *Courtesy Steven Binnick, MD.*

Fig. 29.142 Eruptive vellus hair cysts. *Courtesy Rui Tavares Bello, MD.*

Fig. 29.143 Eruptive vellus hair cysts.

Fig. 29.144 Milia. *Courtesy Steven Binnick, MD.*

Fig. 29.145 Milia en plaque. *Courtesy Steven Binnick, MD.*

Fig. 29.146 Auricular pseudocyst.

Fig. 29.147 Median raphae cyst. *Courtesy Shyam Verma, MBBS, DVD.*

Fig. 29.148 Median raphae cyst. *Courtesy Debabrata Bandyopadhyay.*

Fig. 29.149 Thyroglossal duct cyst.

Melanocytic Nevi and Neoplasms 30

The evaluation of pigmented lesions is one of the most important skill sets in dermatology. The incidence of melanoma continues to increase, and early diagnosis plays a critical role in reducing mortality, morbidity, and the cost of health care. Melanocytic lesions may be distributed anywhere on the body, and certain lesions, such as the so-called *zosteriform lentiginous nevus* follow a segmental blaschkoid distribution, suggesting genetic mosaicism. Most benign lesions are round to oval, relatively small, evenly pigmented, and stable in appearance. In contrast, malignant lesions are often asymmetric with an irregular border, uneven pigmentation, larger diameter, and evolve over time. It should be noted that these concepts apply mainly to primary lesions, as metastatic lesions are often spherical and symmetric in all dimensions. The "ABCDs" of melanoma are a useful tool for education of the lay public, but only serve to identify some lesions of potential concern. They often miss amelanotic, symmetric, and evenly pigmented tumors and do not substitute for a dermatologist's global assessment of the lesion. They should never be used as the sole criteria for biopsy or for referral to a dermatologist.

Dermoscopy allows the physician to see lesion characteristics not visible on routine examination, and confocal microscopy offers the potential for in vivo microscopic imaging of some lesions. Ultimately, though, careful visual examination of the patient's skin remains the key initial step in identifying lesions of concern.

Fig. 30.2 Large nevus spilus.

Fig. 30.1 Nevus spilus.

Fig. 30.3 Widespread unilateral nevus spilus.

Fig. 30.4 Lentigo simplex.

Fig. 30.5 Ink spot lentigo. *Courtesy Steven Binnick, MD.*

Fig. 30.6 Solar lentigo. *Courtesy Steven Binnick, MD.*

Fig. 30.7 Solar lentigines.

Fig. 30.8 Labial melanotic macule. *Courtesy Steven Binnick, MD.*

Fig. 30.9 Vulvar melanosis.

Fig. 30.10 Penile melanosis.

Fig. 30.11 Lentigines in LEOPARD syndrome.

Fig. 30.12 Generalized lentiginosis.

Fig. 30.13 Carney syndrome.

Fig. 30.14 Carney syndrome.

Fig. 30.15 Inherited patterned lentiginosis.

Fig. 30.16 Inherited patterned lentiginosis.

Fig. 30.17 Inherited patterned lentiginosis.

Fig. 30.18 Inherited patterned lentiginosis.

Fig. 30.19 Peutz-Jeghers syndrome. *Courtesy Steven Binnick, MD.*

Fig. 30.20 Peutz-Jeghers syndrome.

Fig. 30.21 Becker nevus.

Fig. 30.22 Becker nevus.

Fig. 30.23 Melanoacanthoma.

Fig. 30.24 Junctional nevi.

Fig. 30.25 Junctional acral nevus.

Fig. 30.26 Longitudinal melanonychia secondary to a junctional nevus.

Fig. 30.27 Intradermal nevi.

Fig. 30.28 Intradermal nevi.

Fig. 30.29 Nevus.

Fig. 30.30 Nevus.

Fig. 30.31 Oral blue nevus.

Fig. 30.32 Ocular nevus.

Fig. 30.33 Large variably pigmented nevus in genital area of a woman.

Fig. 30.34 Large irregular nevus on the breast of a woman. Often nevi in such estrogen-dependent sites are larger. *Courtesy Steven Binnick, MD.*

Fig. 30.35 Halo nevus. *Courtesy Steven Binnick, MD.*

Fig. 30.36 Halo nevi. *Courtesy Steven Binnick, MD.*

Fig. 30.37 Congenital nevus. *Courtesy Steven Binnick, MD.*

Fig. 30.38 Congenital nevus. *Courtesy Steven Binnick, MD.*

Fig. 30.39 Congenital nevus. *Courtesy Steven Binnick, MD.*

Fig. 30.40 Congenital nevus. Note thick hair within the nevus.

Fig. 30.41 Congenital nevus.

Fig. 30.42 Congenital nevus.

Fig. 30.43 Spitz nevus. *Courtesy Steven Binnick, MD.*

Fig. 30.44 Spitz nevus. *Courtesy Steven Binnick, MD.*

Fig. 30.45 Spitz nevus. *Courtesy Curt Samlaska, MD.*

Fig. 30.46 Spindle cell nevi.

Fig. 30.47 Patient with a CDKN2A mutation. This patient had many melanomas and a positive family history of melanoma. *Courtesy Ellen Kim, MD.*

Fig. 30.48 Dysplastic nevi. *Courtesy Michael Ming, MD.*

Fig. 30.49 Dysplastic nevi.

Fig. 30.50 Lentigo maligna.

Fig. 30.51 Lentigo maligna. *Courtesy Steven Binnick, MD.*

Fig. 30.52 Lentigo maligna melanoma.

Fig. 30.54 Superficial spreading melanoma. *Courtesy Steven Binnick, MD.*

Fig. 30.56 Superficial spreading melanoma. *Courtesy Steven Binnick, MD.*

Fig. 30.53 Superficial spreading melanoma. *Courtesy Steven Binnick, MD.*

Fig. 30.55 Superficial spreading melanoma. *Courtesy Steven Binnick, MD.*

Fig. 30.57 Superficial spreading melanoma.

Fig. 30.58 Acral melanoma. *Courtesy Curt Samlaska, MD.*

Fig. 30.59 Acral melanoma. *Courtesy Chris Miller, MD.*

Fig. 30.60 Acral melanoma. *Courtesy Shyam Verma, MBBS, DVD.*

Fig. 30.61 Acral melanoma.

Fig. 30.62 Acral melanoma.

Fig. 30.63 Oral melanoma.

Fig. 30.64 Nodular melanoma. *Courtesy Curt Samlaska, MD.*

Fig. 30.65 Nodular melanoma. *Courtesy Steven Binnick, MD.*

Fig. 30.66 Amelanotic melanoma.

Fig. 30.67 Amelanotic melanoma within a morphea lesion. *Courtesy Curt Samlaska, MD.*

Fig. 30.68 Large melanoma.

Fig. 30.69 Large melanoma.

Fig. 30.70 Satellite metastases from melanoma.

Fig. 30.71 Metastatic melanoma.

Fig. 30.72 Metastatic amelanotic melanoma.

Fig. 30.73 Metastatic melanoma.

Fig. 30.74 Diffuse melanosis in metastatic melanoma; dark hand compared with normal.

Fig. 30.75 Dermal melanocytosis. *Courtesy Steven Binnick, MD.*

Fig. 30.76 Dermal melanocytosis. *Courtesy Steven Binnick, MD.*

Fig. 30.77 Nevus of Ota.

Fig. 30.78 Nevus of Ota. *Courtesy Steven Binnick, MD.*

Fig. 30.79 Nevus of Ota.

Fig. 30.80 Blue nevus.

Fig. 30.81 Blue nevus.

Fig. 30.82 Congenital blue nevus.

Macrophage/Monocyte Disorders 31

This chapter includes granulomatous and histiocytic conditions that are either localized to the skin or can involve the skin as part of a systemic disease. Many will require a skin biopsy to confirm the diagnosis and direct further workup and treatment.

One common granulomatous condition included here is granuloma annulare (GA), a skin condition that typically presents on frictional sites, such as the dorsal feet, forearms, or legs, with skin-colored papules or nodules that form a ring. Other forms of GA can be more difficult to diagnosis, such as the perforating or deep (subcutaneous) forms. Sarcoidosis is another granulomatous condition with skin manifestations in the setting of what is a chronic systemic disease. Skin findings in sarcoidosis can vary and include papules, annular GA-like plaques, ichthyosiform patches, and nodules at site of tattoos. Screening for systemic involvement is essential when sarcoidosis is suspected because it can affect almost every organ in the body.

Histiocytic conditions are featured as well, including juvenile xanthogranulomas (JXG), Langerhans cell histiocytosis (LCH), and rarer conditions such as multicentric reticulohistiocytosis. JXG is a common pediatric condition most commonly limited to the skin in the form of a yellow/orange, smooth papule or nodule. LCH has more varied clinical presentations depending on the age and degree of systemic involvement. Common skin manifestations include erosive, red patches in the folds with petechiae; red-brown papules that can become crusted; xanthomatous nodules; and in adults acneiform eruption on the chest and back.

This portion of the atlas contains images of diseases due to macrophages and monocytes, including granulomatous and histiocytic conditions.

Fig. 31.2 Granuloma annulare. *Courtesy Steven Binnick, MD.*

Fig. 31.1 Granuloma annulare.

Fig. 31.3 Granuloma annulare. *Courtesy Paul Honig, MD.*

Fig. 31.4 Granuloma annulare.

Fig. 31.5 Granuloma annulare.

Fig. 31.6 Granuloma annulare.

Fig. 31.7 Granuloma annulare.

Fig. 31.8 Granuloma annulare.

Fig. 31.9 Granuloma annulare.

Fig. 31.10 Granuloma annulare.

Fig. 31.11 Granuloma annulare.

Fig. 31.12 Granuloma annulare.

Fig. 31.13 Granuloma annulare.

Fig. 31.14 Disseminated granuloma annulare.

Fig. 31.15 Disseminated granuloma annulare.

Fig. 31.16 Disseminated granuloma annulare.

Fig. 31.17 Disseminated granuloma annulare. *Courtesy Curt Samlaska, MD.*

Fig. 31.18 Disseminated granuloma annulare. *Courtesy Curt Samlaska, MD.*

Fig. 31.19 Granuloma annulare.

Fig. 31.20 Perforating granuloma annulare. *Courtesy Curt Samlaska, MD.*

Fig. 31.21 Perforating granuloma annulare. *Courtesy Curt Samlaska, MD.*

Fig. 31.22 Deep granuloma annulare. *Courtesy Ken Greer, MD.*

Fig. 31.23 Subcutaneous granuloma annulare.

Fig. 31.24 Facial granuloma annulare. *Courtesy Steven Binnick, MD.*

Fig. 31.25 Annular elastolytic granuloma.

Fig. 31.26 Annular elastolytic granuloma.

Fig. 31.27 Annular elastolytic granuloma. *Courtesy Curt Samlaska, MD.*

Fig. 31.28 Actinic granuloma.

Fig. 31.29 Miescher granuloma.

Fig. 31.30 Necrobiotic xanthogranuloma.

Fig. 31.31 Necrobiotic xanthogranuloma.

Fig. 31.32 Necrobiotic xanthogranuloma with upper and lower eyelid involvement.

Fig. 31.33 Necrobiotic xanthogranuloma.

Fig. 31.34 Necrobiotic xanthogranuloma.

Fig. 31.35 Papular sarcoidosis. *Courtesy Steven Binnick, MD.*

Fig. 31.36 Papular sarcoidosis.

Fig. 31.37 Papular sarcoidosis.

Fig. 31.38 Papular sarcoidosis.

Fig. 31.39 Papular sarcoidosis.

Fig. 31.40 Papular sarcoidosis.

Fig. 31.41 Nodular sarcoidosis.

Fig. 31.42 Plaque sarcoidosis. *Courtesy Steven Binnick, MD.*

Fig. 31.43 Plaque sarcoidosis. *Courtesy Steven Binnick, MD.*

Fig. 31.44 Plaque sarcoidosis. *Courtesy Steven Binnick, MD.*

Fig. 31.45 Annular sarcoidosis.

Fig. 31.46 Annular genital sarcoid.

Fig. 31.47 Genital sarcoidosis.

Fig. 31.48 Lupus pernio.

Fig. 31.49 Lupus pernio. *Courtesy Steven Binnick, MD.*

Fig. 31.50 Lupus pernio.

Fig. 31.51 Lupus pernio.

Fig. 31.52 Lupus pernio. *Courtesy Steven Binnick, MD.*

Fig. 31.53 Lupus pernio. *Courtesy Steven Binnick, MD.*

Fig. 31.54 Sarcoidosis.

Fig. 31.55 Digital sarcoidosis. *Courtesy Steven Binnick, MD.*

Fig. 31.56 Osseous sarcoidosis. *Courtesy Steven Binnick, MD.*

Fig. 31.57 Hypopigmentation overlying sarcoidosis.

Fig. 31.58 Ulcerative sarcoidosis.

Fig. 31.59 Ulcerative sarcoidosis.

Fig. 31.60 Erythema nodosum–like sarcoidosis. Biopsy was granulomatous.

Fig. 31.61 Sarcoidosis.

Fig. 31.62 Ichthyosiform sarcoidosis. *Courtesy Steven Binnick, MD.*

Fig. 31.63 Ichthyosiform sarcoidosis.

Fig. 31.64 Erythrodermic sarcoidosis.

Fig. 31.65 Erythrodermic sarcoidosis.

Fig. 31.66 Alopecia in sarcoidosis. *Courtesy Misha Rosenbach, MD.*

Fig. 31.67 Sarcoid in a tattoo.

Fig. 31.68 Scar sarcoidosis. *Courtesy Steven Binnick, MD.*

Fig. 31.69 Juvenile xanthogranuloma. *Courtesy Curt Samlaska, MD.*

Fig. 31.70 Juvenile xanthogranuloma. *Courtesy Steven Binnick, MD.*

Fig. 31.71 Juvenile xanthogranuloma.

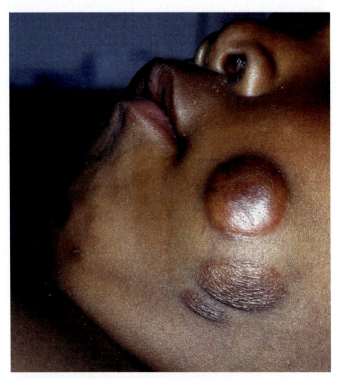

Fig. 31.72 Large juvenile xanthogranuloma.

Fig. 31.73 Multiple juvenile xanthogranuloma. *Courtesy Steven Binnick, MD.*

Fig. 31.74 Juvenile xanthogranulomatous plaque. *Courtesy Scott Norton, MD.*

Fig. 31.75 Benign cephalic histiocytosis. *Courtesy Debabrata Bandyopadhyay, MD.*

Fig. 31.76 Generalized eruptive histiocytomas.

Fig. 31.77 Xanthoma disseminatum. *Courtesy Debabrata Bandyopadhyay, MD.*

Fig. 31.78 Progressive nodular histiocytosis. *Courtesy Scott Norton, MD.*

Fig. 31.79 Progressive nodular histiocytosis.

Fig. 31.80 Reticulohistiocytoma. *Courtesy Steven Binnick, MD.*

Fig. 31.81 Multicentric reticulohistiocytosis.

Fig. 31.82 Multicentric reticulohistiocytosis.

Fig. 31.83 Multicentric reticulohistiocytosis.

Fig. 31.84 Multicentric reticulohistiocytosis.

Fig. 81.85 Multicentric reticulohistiocytosis.

Fig. 31.86 Multicentric reticulohistiocytosis. *Courtesy Steven Binnick, MD.*

Fig. 31.87 Congenital self-healing histiocytomas. *Courtesy Paul Honig, MD.*

Fig. 31.88 Congenital self-healing histiocytomas.

Fig. 31.89 Congenital Langerhans cell histiocytosis.

Fig. 31.90 Congenital Langerhans cell histiocytosis.

Fig. 31.91 Congenital Langerhans cell histiocytosis. *Courtesy Sheilagh Maguiness, MD.*

Fig. 31.92 Langerhans cell histiocytosis.

Fig. 31.93 Langerhans cell histiocytosis.

Fig. 31.94 Langerhans cell histiocytosis. *Courtesy Paul Honig, MD.*

Fig. 31.95 Langerhans cell histiocytosis.

Fig. 31.96 Langerhans cell histiocytosis.

Fig. 31.97 Langerhans cell histiocytosis.

Fig. 31.98 Langerhans cell histiocytosis.

Fig. 31.99 Langerhans cell histiocytosis.

Fig. 31.100 Langerhans cell histiocytosis.

Fig. 31.101 Adult Langerhans cell histiocytosis.

Fig. 31.102 Adult Langerhans cell histiocytosis.

Fig. 31.103 Adult Langerhans cell histiocytosis.

Cutaneous Lymphoid Hyperplasia, Cutaneous T-Cell Lymphoma, Other Malignant Lymphomas, and Allied Diseases

32

The evaluation of lymphoid neoplasms typically requires clinicopathological correlation, and classification often requires panels of immunostains. This section of the atlas will focus on the clinical appearance of cutaneous lymphomas that should prompt the physician to perform a biopsy. The distribution and morphology of the lesion are also helpful in classification of the neoplasm to ensure optimal therapy.

Mycosis fungoides commonly involve the trunk, buttocks, and proximal extremities. The lesions tend to be larger than 5 cm in diameter with a poikilodermatous appearance (mottled, hyperpigmentation and hypopigmentation, atrophy, and telangiectasia). B-cell lymphomas commonly present as plum-colored nodules with a smooth, shiny surface. Discrete nodules on the head and neck, trunk, or proximal extremities; arcuate lesions and nodules on the trunk; taught, shiny nodules on the lower extremities; and multinodular lesions on the legs are all seen in the wide variety of lymphoid neoplasms in this chapter. The lesions of lymphomatoid papulosis are often papulonecrotic, erupt in crops, and resolve spontaneously. Leukemias and myelomas often appear as skin-colored to purple papules and nodules, at times with accompanying hemorrhage into the lesions. This portion of the atlas will focus on the cutaneous manifestations of lymphoid proliferations.

Fig. 32.1 Cutaneous lymphoid hyperplasia, nodular B-cell pattern.

Fig. 32.2 Cutaneous lymphoid hyperplasia, nodular B-cell pattern.

Fig. 32.3 Cutaneous lymphoid hyperplasia, nodular B-cell pattern.

Fig. 32.4 Cutaneous lymphoid hyperplasia, bandlike T-cell pattern.

Fig. 32.5 Jessner lymphocytic infiltrate of the skin.

Fig. 32.7 Mycosis fungoides, patch stage.

Fig. 32.6 Mycosis fungoides, patch stage.

Fig. 32.9 Mycosis fungoides, patch stage.

Fig. 32.8 Mycosis fungoides, patch stage.

Fig. 32.10 Mycosis fungoides, patch stage.

Fig. 32.11 Mycosis fungoides, patch stage.

Fig. 32.12 Mycosis fungoides, patch stage.

Fig. 32.13 Mycosis fungoides, patch stage.

Fig. 32.14 Mycosis fungoides, patch stage.

Fig. 32.15 Mycosis fungoides, patch stage.

Fig. 32.16 Mycosis fungoides, patch stage.

Fig. 32.17 Mycosis fungoides, patch stage. *Courtesy Scott Norton, MD.*

Fig. 32.18 Mycosis fungoides, patch stage with poikiloderma.

Fig. 32.19 Mycosis fungoides, patch stage with poikiloderma. *Courtesy Steven Binnick, MD.*

Fig. 32.20 Mycosis fungoides, patch stage with poikiloderma. *Courtesy Steven Binnick, MD.*

Fig. 32.21 Mycosis fungoides, plaque stage.

Fig. 32.22 Mycosis fungoides, plaque stage.

Fig. 32.23 Mycosis fungoides, plaque stage. *Courtesy Steven Binnick, MD.*

Fig. 32.24 Mycosis fungoides, plaque stage. *Courtesy Steven Binnick, MD.*

Fig. 32.25 Mycosis fungoides, plaque stage. *Courtesy Steven Binnick, MD.*

Fig. 32.26 Mycosis fungoides, tumor stage.

Fig. 32.27 Mycosis fungoides, tumor stage.

Fig. 32.28 Mycosis fungoides, tumor stage. *Courtesy Steven Binnick, MD.*

Fig. 32.29 Mycosis fungoides, tumor stage.

Fig. 32.30 Mycosis fungoides, tumor stage. *Courtesy Maria Hicks, MD.*

Fig. 32.31 Palmar plantar mycosis fungoides.

Fig. 32.32 Palmar plantar mycosis fungoides. *Courtesy Steven Binnick, MD.*

Fig. 32.33 Palmar plantar mycosis fungoides.

Fig. 32.34 Alopecia mucinosa associated with mycosis fungoides. *Courtesy Ellen Kim, MD.*

Fig. 32.35 Follicular mycosis fungoides.

Fig. 32.36 Follicular mycosis fungoides. *Courtesy Ellen Kim, MD.*

Fig. 32.37 Follicular mycosis fungoides. *Courtesy Ellen Kim, MD.*

Fig. 32.38 Follicular mycosis fungoides. *Courtesy Alain Rook, MD.*

Fig. 32.39 Follicular mycosis fungoides with large cell transformation. *Courtesy Alain Rook, MD.*

Fig. 32.40 Sézary syndrome. *Courtesy Alain Rook, MD.*

Fig. 32.41 Sézary syndrome. *Courtesy Alain Rook, MD.*

Fig. 32.42 Sézary syndrome. *Courtesy Ken Greer, MD.*

Fig. 32.43 Sézary syndrome. *Courtesy Ken Greer, MD.*

Fig. 32.44 Sézary syndrome.

Fig. 32.45 Granulomatous slack skin.

Fig. 32.46 Granulomatous slack skin.

Fig. 32.47 Lymphomatoid papulosis.

Fig. 32.48 Lymphomatoid papulosis.

Fig. 32.49 Lymphomatoid papulosis. *Courtesy Alain Rook, MD.*

Fig. 32.50 Lymphomatoid papulosis. *Courtesy Steven Binnick, MD.*

Fig. 32.51 Pityriasis lichenoides et varioliformis acuta.

Fig. 32.52 Pityriasis lichenoides et varioliformis acuta.

Fig. 32.53 Pityriasis lichenoides et varioliformis acuta.

Fig. 32.54 Pityriasis lichenoides et varioliformis acuta. *Courtesy Steven Binnick, MD.*

Fig. 32.55 Ulceronecrotic Mucha-Habermann disease.

Fig. 32.56 Pityriasis lichenoides chronica.

Fig. 32.57 Pityriasis lichenoides chronica.

Fig. 32.58 Pityriasis lichenoides chronica.

Fig. 32.59 Pityriasis lichenoides chronica.

Fig. 32.60 CD30+ anaplastic T-cell lymphoma. *Courtesy Alain Rook, MD.*

Fig. 32.61 CD30+ anaplastic T-cell lymphoma. *Courtesy Alain Rook, MD.*

Fig. 32.62 Gamma-delta T-cell lymphoma. *Courtesy Ellen Kim, MD.*

Fig. 32.63 Gamma-delta T-cell lymphoma. *Courtesy Alain Rook, MD.*

Fig. 32.64 Gamma-delta T-cell lymphoma. *Courtesy Alain Rook, MD.*

Fig. 32.65 Subcutaneous T-cell lymphoma.

Fig. 32.66 Natural killer T-cell lymphoma. *Courtesy Alain Rook, MD.*

Fig. 32.67 Hydroa vacciniforme–like natural killer T-cell lymphoma.

Fig. 32.68 Hydroa vacciniforme–like natural killer T-cell lymphoma.

Fig. 32.69 B-cell lymphoma.

Fig. 32.70 B-cell lymphoma.

Fig. 32.71 B-cell lymphoma.

Fig. 32.72 B-cell lymphoma.

Fig. 32.73 Secondary cutaneous lymphoma.

Fig. 32.74 B-cell lymphoma, leg type.

Fig. 32.75 Plasmacytomas.

Fig. 32.76 Plasmacytomas.

Fig. 32.77 Malignant histiocytosis.

Fig. 32.78 Acute myelomonocytic leukemia cutis.

Fig. 32.79 Acute myelomonocytic leukemia cutis.

Fig. 32.80 Leukemia cutis.

Fig. 32.81 Acute myelogenous leukemia cutis.

Fig. 32.82 Acute myelomonocytic leukemia.

Fig. 32.83 Leukemia cutis.

Fig. 32.84 Leukemia cutis. *Courtesy Robert Micheletti, MD.*

Fig. 32.85 Leukemia cutis. *Courtesy Robert Micheletti, MD.*

Fig. 32.86 Hypereosinophilic syndrome. *Courtesy John Stanley, MD.*

Fig. 32.87 Angioimmunoblastic T-cell lymphoma.

Fig. 32.88 Rosai-Dorfman disease.

Fig. 32.89 Rosai-Dorfman disease. *Courtesy Curt Samlaska, MD.*

Diseases of Skin Appendages 33

The field of dermatology includes diseases of both skin and the skin appendages, namely hair, sweat glands, and nails. A great variety of conditions affect the skin appendages, and some are isolated to the hair, nail, or sweat glands, whereas some are found in the setting of a more widespread cutaneous or systemic disease.

Diseases of the hair include alopecia, hirsutism, and those affecting the hair color and hair shaft. Evaluation of these conditions includes a directed history along with evaluation of the scalp, eyebrows, eyelashes, and body hair. Beyond a biopsy of the affected region to assess the hair follicles, bedside tests such as the pull test and tug test help investigate the integrity of the hair follicles and shafts, respectively.

Examination of the nail units includes inspection of the nail plate, nail folds, and cuticles, as well as the nail bed and lunula. Like hair conditions, some nail conditions are isolated to the nail, such as melanonychia, and others are associated with more widespread disease. Some nail findings can be a clue to an underlying skin condition, such as the pitting seen in psoriasis, whereas other nail findings can be associated with systemic diseases such as half-and-half nails with proximal white discoloration that can be seen in patients with kidney disease. Still other nail conditions can be secondary to medications or trauma.

Lastly, sweat glands include the widespread eccrine glands and more localized apocrine variant predominantly found in the axillae and groin. This portion of the atlas will provide images of those conditions involving the skin appendages, including the hair, sweat glands, and nails.

Fig. 33.2 Alopecia areata.

Fig. 33.1 Alopecia areata.

Fig. 33.3 Alopecia areata.

Fig. 33.4 Alopecia areata of the beard.

Fig. 33.5 Ophiasis type of alopecia areata. *Courtesy Steven Binnick, MD.*

Fig. 33.6 Alopecia universalis.

Fig. 33.7 Alopecia universalis.

Fig. 33.8 Recurrent alopecia areata in an atopic patient.

Fig. 33.9 Alopecia areata in a Down syndrome patient.

Fig. 33.10 Nails of a patient with alopecia areata. *Courtesy Steven Binnick, MD.*

Fig. 33.11 Nails of a patient with alopecia areata. *Courtesy Steven Binnick, MD.*

Fig. 33.12 Loose anagen hair syndrome.

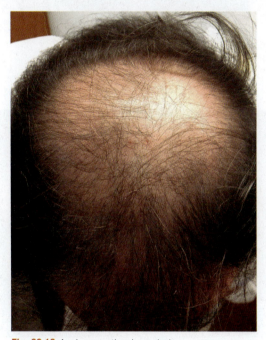

Fig. 33.13 Androgenetic alopecia in a man. *Courtesy Len Sperling, MD.*

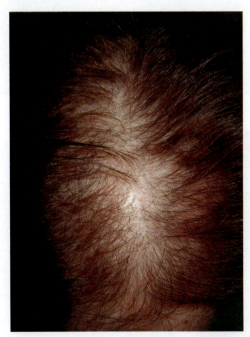

Fig. 33.14 Androgenetic alopecia in a woman. *Courtesy Len Sperling, MD.*

Fig. 33.15 Trichotillosis.

Fig. 33.16 Trichotillosis.

Fig. 33.17 Alopecia mucinosa.

Fig. 33.18 Alopecia mucinosa.

Fig. 33.19 Congenital triangular alopecia.

Fig. 33.20 Discoid lupus of the scalp.

Fig. 33.21 Scarring alopecia secondary to discoid lupus erythematosus. *Courtesy Steven Binnick, MD.*

Fig. 33.22 Lichen planopilaris.

Fig. 33.23 Frontal fibrosing alopecia. *Courtesy Len Sperling, MD.*

Fig. 33.24 Frontal fibrosing alopecia.

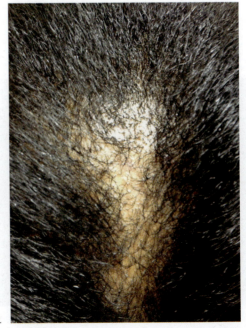

Fig. 33.25 Central centrifugal cicatricial alopecia. *Courtesy Len Sperling, MD.*

Fig. 33.26 Central centrifugal cicatricial alopecia. *Courtesy Len Sperling, MD.*

Fig. 33.27 Folliculitis decalvans.

Fig. 33.28 Erosive pustular dermatitis of the scalp.

Fig. 33.29 Tufted folliculitis.

Fig. 33.30 Pseudopelade of Brocq. *Courtesy Steven Binnick, MD.*

Fig. 33.31 Traction alopecia.

Fig. 33.32 Traction alopecia.

Fig. 33.33 Alopecia neoplastica from metastatic breast cancer.

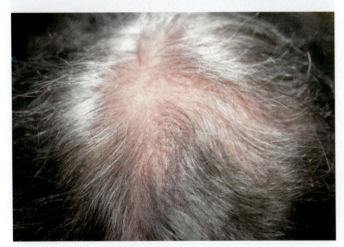

Fig. 33.34 Keratosis follicularis spinulosa decalvans. *Courtesy Steven Binnick, MD.*

Fig. 33.35 Atrichia with papular lesions. *Courtesy Steven Binnick, MD.*

Fig. 33.36 Atrichia with papular lesions.

Fig. 33.37 Poliosis. *Courtesy Steven Binnick, MD.*

Fig. 33.38 Flag sign.

Fig. 33.39 Pili torti. *Courtesy Curt Samlaska, MD.*

Fig. 33.40 Pili torti. *Courtesy Curt Samlaska, MD.*

Fig. 33.41 Menkes kinky hair syndrome. *Courtesy Paul Honig, MD.*

Fig. 33.42 Menkes kinky hair syndrome.

Fig. 33.43 Proximal trichorrhexis nodosa.

Fig. 33.44 Trichorrhexis invaginata in Netherton syndrome.

Fig. 33.45 Pili annulati.

Fig. 33.46 Monilethrix.

Fig. 33.47 Monilethrix.

Fig. 33.48 Uncombable hair syndrome. *Courtesy Paul Honig, MD.*

Fig. 33.49 Uncombable hair syndrome.

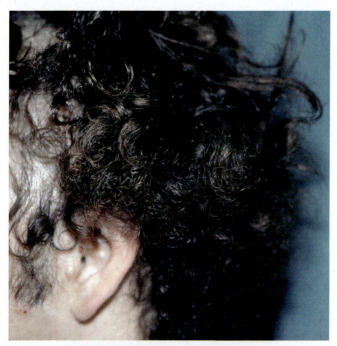

Fig. 33.50 Progressive kinking of the hair. *Courtesy Ken Greer, MD.*

Fig. 33.51 Wooly hair.

Fig. 33.53 Pseudofolliculitis barbae. *Courtesy Steven Binnick, MD.*

Fig. 33.52 Pseudofolliculitis barbae. *Courtesy Steven Binnick, MD.*

Fig. 33.54 Pili multigemini.

Fig. 33.55 Trichostasis spinulosa. *Courtesy Steven Binnick, MD.*

Fig. 33.56 Hypertrichosis cubiti. *Courtesy Paul Honig, MD.*

Fig. 33.57 Localized hypertrichosis over the sacrum with a lipoma and underlying tethered cord.

Fig. 33.58 Hypertrichosis from minoxidil. *Courtesy Paul Honig, MD.*

Fig. 33.59 Hirsutism and acne. *Courtesy Steven Binnick, MD.*

Fig. 33.60 Hirsutism and acne. *Courtesy Steven Binnick, MD.*

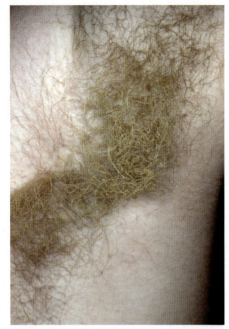

Fig. 33.61 Trichomycosis axillaris. *Courtesy Steven Binnick, MD.*

Fig. 33.62 Trichomycosis axillaris.

Fig. 33.63 Tinea amiantacea. *Courtesy Scott Norton, MD.*

Fig. 33.64 Disseminate and recurrent infundibulofolliculitis.

Fig. 33.65 Disseminate and recurrent infundibulofolliculitis.

Fig. 33.66 Palmar hyperhidrosis.

Fig. 33.67 Fox-Fordyce disease.

Fig. 33.68 Fox-Fordyce disease. *Courtesy Steven Binnick, MD.*

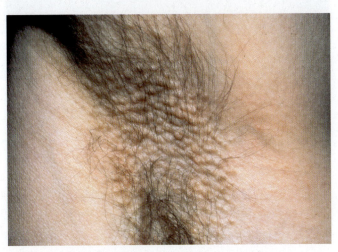

Fig. 33.69 Fox-Fordyce disease with xanthomatous change.

Fig. 33.70 Perforating disorder of renal failure. *Courtesy Scott Norton, MD.*

Fig. 33.71 Reactive perforating collagenosis.

Fig. 33.72 Nail lichen planus. *Courtesy Adam Rubin, MD.*

Fig. 33.73 Nail lichen planus.

Fig. 33.74 Nail lichen planus.

Fig. 33.75 Oil spot in a psoriatic nail.

Fig. 33.76 Nail pits in psoriatic nails.

Fig. 33.77 Hyperkeratosis in a psoriatic nail. Patient also has psoriatic arthritis.

Fig. 33.78 Nail psoriasis in a patient with psoriatic arthritis.

Fig. 33.79 Darier disease of the nail.

Fig. 33.80 Clubbing.

Fig. 33.81 Clubbing.

Fig. 33.82 Clubbing.

Fig. 33.83 Koilonychia with trachyonychia. *Courtesy Adam Rubin, MD.*

Fig. 33.84 Koilonychia.

Fig. 33.85 Congenital onychodysplasia of the index finger.

Fig. 33.86 Congenital onychodysplasia of the index finger.

Fig. 33.87 Trachyonychia. *Courtesy Adam Rubin, MD.*

Fig. 33.88 Trachyonychia. *Courtesy Adam Rubin, MD.*

Fig. 33.89 Anonychia.

Fig. 33.90 Onychogryphosis. *Courtesy Scott Norton, MD.*

Fig. 33.91 Onychomadesis after hand-foot-mouth disease.

Fig. 33.92 Onychomadesis after toxic epidermal necrolysis.

Fig. 33.93 Beau lines. *Courtesy Steven Binnick, MD.*

Fig. 33.94 Half-and-half nails.

Fig. 33.95 Muehrcke lines.

Fig. 33.96 Mee lines.

Fig. 33.97 Terry nail.

Fig. 33.99 Racquet nails. *Courtesy Adam Rubin, MD.*

Fig. 33.101 Nail patella syndrome with nail dystrophy.

Fig. 33.98 Onychoschizia.

Fig. 33.100 Nail patella syndrome. Note triangular lunulae.

Fig. 33.102 Onychophagia.

Fig. 33.103 Nail dystrophy, with washboard nail due to habit of pushing back cuticle. *Courtesy Steven Binnick, MD.*

Fig. 33.104 Onycholysis. *Courtesy Steven Binnick, MD.*

Fig. 33.105 Median nail dystrophy. *Courtesy Steven Binnick, MD.*

Fig. 33.106 Median nail dystrophy.

Fig. 33.107 Pterygium unguis. *Courtesy Adam Rubin, MD.*

Fig. 33.108 Pterygium inversum unguis. *Courtesy Adam Rubin, MD.*

Fig. 33.109 Pincer nail.

Fig. 33.110 Retronychia. *Courtesy Rui Tavares Bello, MD.*

Fig. 33.111 Leukonychia. *Courtesy Scott Norton, MD.*

Fig. 33.112 Transverse leukonychia. *Courtesy Curt Samlaska, MD.*

Fig. 33.113 Erythronychia in Darier disease. *Courtesy Steven Binnick, MD.*

Fig. 33.114 Melanonychia striata, benign, involved multiple nails in this African American patient.

Fig. 33.115 Melanonychia striata, benign.

Fig. 33.116 Melanonychia striata caused by melanoma in situ. *Courtesy Adam Rubin, MD.*

Fig. 33.117 Transverse nail bands secondary to chemotherapy.

Fig. 33.118 Zidovudine pigmentation.

Fig. 33.119 Zidovudine pigmentation.

Fig. 33.120 Green nail.

Fig. 33.121 Exogenous nail staining. Note pigment follows the curvature of the proximal and lateral nail folds.

Fig. 33.122 Red lunula.

Fig. 33.123 Spotted lunula.

Fig. 33.124 Subungual hematoma.

Fig. 33.125 Splinter hemorrhage. *Courtesy Steven Binnick, MD.*

Fig. 33.126 Yellow nail syndrome. *Courtesy Adam Rubin, MD.*

Fig. 33.127 Yellow nail syndrome.

Fig. 33.128 Yellow nail syndrome.

Fig. 33.129 Onychopapilloma. *Courtesy Adam Rubin, MD.*

Fig. 33.130 Onychomatricoma. *Courtesy Adam Rubin, MD.*

Fig. 33.131 Bowen disease of the nail bed.

Fig. 33.132 Squamous cell carcinoma.

Fig. 33.133 Melanoma.

Fig. 33.134 Melanoma.

Diseases of Mucous Membranes   34

Diseases of the mucous membranes include those involving the lips, tongue, palate, gingiva, teeth, and the floor of the mouth. Inspection of this entire surface should be included in the full skin examination to screen for evidence of mucocutaneous conditions, such as lichen planus, and primary diseases of the mucosa, such as squamous cell carcinoma of the lip. Routine examination of these surfaces also allows one to become familiar with the spectrum of benign findings such as many forms of oral melanosis.

Primary conditions of the mucosal surfaces include changes to the tongue, such as median rhomboid glossitis or inflammation of the taste buds known as *papillitis*. Aphthous ulcers provide another example of a primary oral disease, and they are featured here with their classic round, shallow, white ulcers with surrounding bright red rims.

Many oral findings can be found in the setting of a systemic disease such as inflammatory bowel disease (IBD). In IBD there are several related mucosal diseases, including the cobblestoned appearance of the mucosa, oral ulcers, granulomatous cheilitis, and pyostomatitis vegetans. Nutritional deficiencies, fixed drug eruptions, and Behçet syndrome are examples of other systemic diseases with important mucosal findings.

This portion of the atlas includes images of many common and uncommon findings of import that may be seen upon examination of the mucosal membranes.

Fig. 34.1 Allergic contact cheilitis to topical steroids. *Courtesy Glen Crawford, MD.*

Fig. 34.2 Actinic cheilitis. *Courtesy Joseph Sobanko, MD.*

Fig. 34.3 Actinic cheilitis. *Courtesy Joseph Sobanko, MD.*

Fig. 34.4 Cheilitis secondary to lip licking. *Courtesy Steven Binnick, MD.*

Fig. 34.5 Postinflammatory hypopigmentation secondary to lip licking. *Courtesy Scott Norton, MD.*

Fig. 34.6 Cheilitis glandularis. *Courtesy Debabrata Bandyopadhyay, MD.*

Fig. 34.7 Cheilitis glandularis with leukoplakia.

Fig. 34.8 Angular cheilitis. *Courtesy Steven Binnick, MD.*

Fig. 34.9 Angular cheilitis.

Fig. 34.10 Plasma cell cheilitis.

Fig. 34.11 Cutaneous Crohn disease. *Courtesy Curt Samlaska, MD.*

Fig. 34.12 Cutaneous Crohn disease.

Fig. 34.13 Cutaneous Crohn disease.

Fig. 34.14 Cutaneous Crohn disease. *Courtesy Curt Samlaska, MD.*

Fig. 34.15 Cutaneous Crohn disease.

Fig. 34.16 Cutaneous Crohn disease.

Fig. 34.17 Oral Crohn disease. *Courtesy Curt Samlaska, MD.*

Fig. 34.18 Oral Crohn disease. *Courtesy Curt Samlaska, MD.*

Fig. 34.19 Pyostomatitis vegetans. *Courtesy Scott Norton, MD.*

Fig. 34.20 Pyostomatitis vegetans. *Courtesy Scott Norton, MD.*

Fig. 34.21 Granulomatous cheilitis.

Fig. 34.22 Melkersson-Rosenthal syndrome.

Fig. 34.23 Melkersson-Rosenthal syndrome.

Fig. 34.24 Fordyce spots.

Fig. 34.25 Nicotine stomatitis. *Courtesy Ken Greer, MD.*

Fig. 34.26 Torus palatinus.

Fig. 34.27 Torus mandibularis.

Fig. 34.28 Fissured tongue.

Fig. 34.29 Fissured tongue. *Courtesy Steven Binnick, MD.*

Fig. 34.30 Geographic tongue. *Courtesy Ken Greer, MD.*

Fig. 34.31 Geographic tongue. *Courtesy Steven Binnick, MD.*

Fig. 34.32 Annulus migrans.

Fig. 34.33 Black hairy tongue. *Courtesy Steven Binnick, MD.*

Fig. 34.34 Black hairy tongue. *Courtesy Steven Binnick, MD.*

Fig. 34.35 Median rhomboid glossitis. *Courtesy Steven Binnick, MD.*

Fig. 34.36 Median rhomboid glossitis. *Courtesy Steven Binnick, MD.*

Fig. 34.37 Cutaneous dental sinus.

Fig. 34.38 Poor oral hygiene in the patient shown in Fig. 34.37.

Fig. 34.39 Cutaneous dental sinus.

Fig. 34.40 Cutaneous dental sinus. *Courtesy Steven Binnick, MD.*

Fig. 34.41 Leukoplakia.

Fig. 34.42 Leukoplakia. *Courtesy Steven Binnick, MD.*

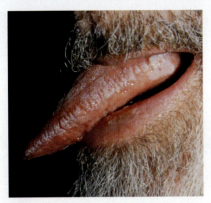

Fig. 34.43 Oral hairy leukoplakia.

Fig. 34.44 Oral florid papillomatosis. *Courtesy Steven Binnick, MD.*

Fig. 34.45 Oral florid papillomatosis. *Courtesy Steven Binnick, MD.*

Fig. 34.46 Proliferative verrucous leukoplakia.

Fig. 34.47 Squamous cell carcinoma secondary to chewing betel nut. *Courtesy Shyam Verma, MBBS, DVD.*

Fig. 34.48 Squamous cell carcinoma.

Fig. 34.49 Squamous cell carcinoma.

Fig. 34.50 Squamous cell carcinoma.

Fig. 34.51 Acquired dyskeratotic leukoplakia.

Fig. 34.52 Acquired dyskeratotic leukoplakia, gingiva.

Fig. 34.53 Acquired dyskeratotic leukoplakia, genital involvement.

Fig. 34.54 White sponge nevus.

Fig. 34.55 White sponge nevus.

Fig. 34.56 Physiologic pigmentation.

Fig. 34.57 Physiologic oral pigmentation. *Courtesy Scott Norton, MD.*

Fig. 34.58 Physiologic oral pigmentation.

Fig. 34.59 Oral nevus.

Fig. 34.60 Melanoma.

Fig. 34.61 Oral melanotic macule.

Fig. 34.62 Oral melanotic macule.

Fig. 34.63 Oral melanotic macule.

Fig. 34.64 Chloroquine hyperpigmentation.

Fig. 34.65 Chlorpromazine hyperpigmentation.

Fig. 34.66 Minocycline hyperpigmentation.

Fig. 34.67 Oat cell carcinoma–associated pigmentation.

Fig. 34.68 Amalgam tattoo.

Fig. 34.69 Oral melanosis.

Fig. 34.70 Oral melanosis with progressive involvement.

Fig. 34.71 Epulis.

Fig. 34.72 Pyogenic granuloma.

Fig. 34.73 Pyogenic granuloma.

Fig. 34.74 Mucocele.

Fig. 34.75 Mucocele.

Fig. 34.76 Ranula.

Fig. 34.77 Ranula. *Courtesy Steven Binnick, MD.*

Fig. 34.78 Ranula. *Courtesy Steven Binnick, MD.*

Fig. 34.79 Acute necrotizing ulcerative gingivostomatitis. *Courtesy Department of Oral Medicine, University of Pennsylvania School of Dentistry.*

Fig. 34.80 Noma.

Fig. 34.81 Noma.

Fig. 34.82 Aphthous stomatitis. *Courtesy Steven Binnick, MD.*

Fig. 34.83 Aphthous stomatitis.

Fig. 34.84 Aphthous stomatitis. *Courtesy Steven Binnick, MD.*

Fig. 34.85 Aphthous stomatitis. *Courtesy Steven Binnick, MD.*

Fig. 34.86 Major aphthous stomatitis.

Fig. 34.87 Major aphthous stomatitis.

Fig. 34.88 Behçet disease. *Courtesy Ken Greer, MD.*

Fig. 34.89 Behçet disease.

Fig. 34.90 Behçet disease. *Courtesy Ken Greer, MD.*

Fig. 34.91 Behçet disease.

Fig. 34.92 Behçet disease.

Cutaneous Vascular Diseases 35

This section of the atlas will focus on vascular disorders of the skin, including such entities as Raynaud disease, erythromelalgia, livedo racemosa, livedoid vasculopathy, cryoglobulinemia, purpura fulminans, superficial thrombophlebitis, purpura, and vasculitis. As with other disorders of skin, the color, morphology, and distribution of skin lesions are critical to establishment of an accurate diagnosis. Immune complex–mediated disease often affects dependent areas of skin, whereas embolic and vasoconstrictive phenomena affect acral sites. Diseases affecting the post–capillary venule or capillaries seldom result in cutaneous necrosis and tend to produce lesions with a round-to-oval configuration, whereas diseases affecting arterioles commonly result in angular stellate infarcts and retiform purpura. Postcapillary venule disease results in petichiae, or palpable or macular areas of purpura, whereas chronic capillaritis presents with hemosiderin staining and thumbprint, annular, eczematous, or lichenoid-containing petechiae. Forms of vasculitis associated with a stellate or retiform morphology include antineutrophil cytoplasmic antibody–associated vasculitis, rheumatoid vasculitis, and septic vasculitis. Ischemic disease is often associated with pain, and severe or prolonged ischemia results in necrosis. Vasodilatation may relate to temperature regulation, abnormal shunting of blood, or small-fiber neuropathy, as in the case of erythromelalgia. The morphology and distribution of the lesions suggest the correct site and appropriate depth for a biopsy.

Fig. 35.2 Raynaud phenomenon with digital ulcers.

Fig. 35.1 Raynaud phenomenon secondary to mixed connective tissue disease.

Fig. 35.3 Erythromelalgia.

Fig. 35.4 Erythromelalgia.

Fig. 35.5 Livedo reticularis.

Fig. 35.6 Livedo reticularis caused by amantadine.

Fig. 35.7 Livedo racemosa.

Fig. 35.8 Livedo racemosa. *Courtesy Rui Tavares Bello, MD.*

Fig. 35.9 Sneddon syndrome.

Fig. 35.10 Necrotizing livedo.

Fig. 35.11 Purple toe secondary to cholesterol emboli.

Fig. 35.12 Cholesterol emboli. *Courtesy Curt Samlaska, MD.*

Fig. 35.13 Cholesterol emboli.

Fig. 35.14 Livedoid vasculopathy.

Fig. 35.15 Atrophy blanche.

Fig. 35.16 Calciphylaxis.

Fig. 35.17 Calciphylaxis.

Fig. 35.18 Purpura in old age.

Fig. 35.19 Purpura in old age.

Fig. 35.20 Purpura in old age.

Fig. 35.21 Immune thrombocytopenic purpura.

Fig. 35.22 Immune thrombocytopenic purpura.

Fig. 35.23 Thrombotic thrombocytopenic purpura.

Fig. 35.24 Thrombotic thrombocytopenic purpura.

Fig. 35.25 Cryoglobulinemic vasculitis. *Courtesy Robert Micheletti, MD.*

Fig. 35.26 Waldenström hypergammaglobulinemic purpura.

Fig. 35.27 Purpura fulminans.

Fig. 35.28 Purpura fulminans.

Fig. 35.29 Homozygous protein C deficiency.

Fig. 35.30 Protein S deficiency.

Fig. 35.31 Catastrophic antiphospholipid antibody syndrome.

Fig. 35.32 Superficial thrombophlebitis.

Fig. 35.33 Migrating superficial thrombophlebitis.

Fig. 35.34 Mondor disease.

Fig. 35.35 Purpura from coin rubbing. *Courtesy Steven Binnick, MD.*

Fig. 35.36 Racquetball-induced purpura.

Fig. 35.37 Purpura after vomiting. *Courtesy Steven Binnick, MD.*

Fig. 35.38 Cough-induced purpura.

Fig. 35.39 Passion purpura.

Fig. 35.40 Psychogenic purpura. *Courtesy Steven Binnick, MD.*

Fig. 35.41 Psychogenic purpura. *Courtesy Steven Binnick, MD.*

Fig. 35.42 Schamberg disease.

Fig. 35.43 Purpura annularis telangiectodes.

Fig. 35.44 Lichen aureus.

Fig. 35.45 Leukocytoclastic vasculitis.

Fig. 35.46 Leukocytoclastic vasculitis.

Fig. 35.47 Leukocytoclastic vasculitis.

Fig. 35.48 Leukocytoclastic vasculitis. *Courtesy Steven Binnick, MD.*

Fig. 35.49 Leukocytoclastic vasculitis.

Fig. 35.50 Henoch-Schönlein purpura. *Courtesy Steven Binnick, MD.*

Fig. 35.51 Henoch-Schönlein purpura.

Fig. 35.52 Henoch-Schönlein purpura.

Fig. 35.53 Henoch-Schönlein purpura. Note lesions at site of pressure.

Fig. 35.54 Adult Henoch-Schönlein purpura.

Fig. 35.55 Acute hemorrhagic edema of infancy.

Fig. 35.56 Acute hemorrhagic edema of infancy.

Fig. 35.57 Acute hemorrhagic edema of infancy.

Fig. 35.58 Urticarial vasculitis.

Fig. 35.59 Urticarial vasculitis.

Fig. 35.60 Urticarial vasculitis.

Fig. 35.61 Cryoglobulinemic vasculitis.

Fig. 35.62 Cryoglobulemic vasculitis.

Fig. 35.63 Erythema elevatum diutinum.

Fig. 35.64 Erythema elevatum diutinum.

Fig. 35.65 Erythema elevatum diutinum.

Fig. 35.66 Erythema elevatum diutinum.

Fig. 35.67 Erythema elevatum diutinum.

Fig. 35.68 Granuloma faciale. *Courtesy Steven Binnick, MD.*

Fig. 35.69 Granuloma faciale. *Courtesy Steven Binnick, MD.*

Fig. 35.70 Granuloma faciale. *Courtesy Steven Binnick, MD.*

Fig. 35.71 Granuloma faciale.

Fig. 35.72 Polyarteritis nodosa.

Fig. 35.73 Polyarteritis nodosa.

Fig. 35.74 Polyarteritis nodosa.

Fig. 35.75 Polyarteritis nodosa.

Fig. 35.76 Drug-induced antineutrophil cytoplasmic antibody–positive vasculitis. *Courtesy Robert Micheletti, MD.*

Fig. 35.77 Granulomatosis with polyangiitis. *Courtesy Campbell Stewart, MD.*

Fig. 35.78 Granulomatosis with polyangiitis. *Courtesy Campbell Stewart, MD.*

Fig. 35.79 Granulomatosis with polyangiitis.

Fig. 35.80 Granulomatosis with polyangiitis.

Fig. 35.81 Granulomatosis with polyangiitis.

Fig. 35.82 Urticarial plaques in a patient with eosinophilic granulomatosis with polyangitis. *Courtesy Robert Micheletti, MD.*

Fig. 35.83 Eosinophilic granulomatosis with polyangiitis. *Courtesy Robert Micheletti, MD.*

Fig. 35.84 Eosinophilic granulomatosis with polyangiitis. *Courtesy Robert Micheletti, MD.*

Fig. 35.85 Levamisole-induced vasculopathy. *Courtesy Antoine Sreih, MD.*

Fig. 35.86 Levamisole-induced vasculopathy. *Courtesy Misha Rosenbach, MD.*

Fig. 35.87 Levamisole-induced vasculopathy. *Courtesy Misha Rosenbach, MD.*

Fig. 35.88 Temporal arteritis.

Fig. 35.89 Degos disease. *Courtesy Robert Micheletti, MD.*

Fig. 35.90 Degos disease. *Courtesy Robert Micheletti, MD.*

Fig. 35.91 Buerger disease.

Fig. 35.92 Buerger disease.

Fig. 35.93 Buerger disease.

Fig. 35.94 Arteriosclerosis obliterans.

Fig. 35.95 Kawasaki disease.

Fig. 35.96 Kawasaki disease.

Fig. 35.97 Kawasaki disease.

Fig. 35.98 Kawasaki disease.

Fig. 35.99 Kawasaki disease.

Fig. 35.100 Kawasaki disease.

Fig. 35.101 Kawasaki disease.

Fig. 35.102 Kawasaki disease.

Fig. 35.103 Kawasaki disease.

Fig. 35.104 Generalized essential telangiectasia.

Fig. 35.105 Cutaneous collagenous vasculopathy.

Fig. 35.106 Unilateral nevoid telangiectasia.

Fig. 35.107 Osler-Weber-Rendu disease.

Fig. 35.108 Osler-Weber-Rendu disease.

Fig. 35.109 Osler-Weber-Rendu disease.

Fig. 35.110 Osler-Weber-Rendu disease.

Fig. 35.111 Osler-Weber-Rendu disease.

Fig. 35.112 Stasis dermatitis.

Fig. 35.113 Stasis dermatitis with early ulceration.

Fig. 35.114 Stasis dermatitis.

Fig. 35.115 Stasis dermatitis with ulceration.

Fig. 35.116 Arterial ulceration.

Fig. 35.117 Obesity-related lymphedema.

Disturbances of Pigmentation   36

Pigmentary disorders of the skin may present with depigmentation, hypopigmentation, or hyperpigmentation. The color, morphology, and distribution of the lesions help to suggest the correct diagnosis. Vitiligo may be segmental (blaschkoid), acral (lips and tips), or truncal in distribution. Each presentation has implications for treatment. The lesions of vitiligo must be distinguished from those of pityriasis alba, hypopigmented mycosis fungoides, leprosy, and the confetti-like depigmentation and ash-leaf macules of tuberous sclerosis. Hyperpigmented lesions cover a similar spectrum of disorders from lichenoid dermatoses to melasma and the café-au-lait macules of neurofibromatosis. This section of the atlas will focus on disorders of pigmentation not found in other chapters of the book, including vitiligo, piebaldism, pigmentary demarcation lines, melasma, and Galli-Galli disease. A Wood's lamp is of value in these disorders, as accentuation of the pigment suggests epidermal pigment alternation, whereas a decrease in the appearance of the pigmentary anomaly suggests dermal pigment deposition. Topical treatments can address many forms of epidermal dyspigmentation, whereas laser treatment is often more appropriate for the treatment of dermal pigment. When the clinical examination fails to provide a specific diagnosis, addition of a directed history or biopsy may be required. Fontana staining indicates the presence of melanin, and immunostains such as Mart-1 and Sox-10 confirm the pattern and distribution of melanocytes within the lesion.

Fig. 36.2 Type B pigmentary demarcation.

Fig. 36.1 Type A pigmentary demarcation.

Fig. 36.3 Type C pigmentary demarcation.

Fig. 36.4 Postinflammatory dyspigmentation secondary to lupus erythematosus.

Fig. 36.5 Postinflammatory hyperpigmentation. *Courtesy Steven Binnick, MD.*

Fig. 36.6 Melasma.

Fig. 36.7 Melasma.

Fig. 36.8 Melasma.

Fig. 36.9 Dyschromatosis symmetrica hereditaria. *Courtesy Department of Dermatology, Keio University, School of Medicine, Tokyo, Japan.*

Fig. 36.10 Dyschromatosis symmetrica hereditaria. *Courtesy Department of Dermatology, Keio University, School of Medicine, Tokyo, Japan.*

Fig. 36.11 Dyschromatosis symmetrica hereditaria. *Courtesy Department of Dermatology, Keio University, School of Medicine, Tokyo, Japan.*

Fig. 36.12 Dyschromatosis symmetrica hereditaria. *Courtesy Department of Dermatology, Keio University, School of Medicine, Tokyo, Japan.*

Fig. 36.13 Galli-Galli disease.

Fig. 36.14 Galli-Galli disease.

Fig. 36.15 Galli-Galli disease.

Fig. 36.16 Reticulate acropigmentation of Kitamura. *Courtesy Department of Dermatology, Keio University, School of Medicine, Tokyo, Japan.*

Fig. 36.17 Reticulate acropigmentation of Kitamura. *Courtesy Department of Dermatology, Keio University, School of Medicine, Tokyo, Japan.*

Fig. 36.18 Dermatopathia pigmentosa reticularis.

Fig. 36.19 Dermatopathia pigmentosa reticularis.

Fig. 36.20 Dermatopathia pigmentosa reticularis.

Fig. 36.21 Dyschromatosis universalis hereditaria. *Courtesy Vasanop Vachiramon, MD.*

Fig. 36.22 Dyschromatosis universalis hereditaria. *Courtesy Vasanop Vachiramon, MD.*

Fig. 36.23 Familial progressive hypopigmentation and hyperpigmentation (KITLG mutation). *Courtesy of Lara Wine-Lee, MD, PhD.*

Fig. 36.24 Familial progressive hypopigmentation and hyperpigmentation (KITLG mutation). *Courtesy Lara Wine-Lee, MD, PhD.*

Fig. 36.25 Familial progressive hypopigmentation and hyperpigmentation (KITLG mutation). *Courtesy Lara Wine-Lee, MD, PhD.*

Fig. 36.26 Transient neonatal pustular melanosis.

Fig. 36.27 Transient neonatal pustular melanosis.

Fig. 36.28 Transient neonatal pustular melanosis.

Fig. 36.29 Peutz-Jeghers syndrome.

Fig. 36.30 Laugier-Hunziker syndrome.

Fig. 36.31 Carney syndrome.

Fig. 36.32 Pigmentary changes from arsenic.

Fig. 36.33 Segmental vitiligo.

Fig. 36.35 Vitiligo.

Fig. 36.37 Vitiligo. *Courtesy Steven Binnick, MD.*

Fig. 36.34 Vitiligo.

Fig. 36.36 Vitiligo.

Fig. 36.38 Vitiligo.

Disturbances of pigmentation

Fig. 36.39 Vitiligo.

Fig. 36.40 Vitiligo. *Courtesy Steven Binnick, MD.*

Fig. 36.41 Vitiligo.

Fig. 36.42 Vitiligo.

Fig. 36.43 Vitiligo with koebnerization.

Fig. 36.44 Trichrome vitiligo. *Courtesy Scott Norton, MD.*

Fig. 36.45 Vitiligo.

Fig. 36.46 Poliosis in vitiligo.

Fig. 36.47 Poliosis.

Fig. 36.48 Phenolic depigmentation.

Fig. 36.49 Depigmentation secondary to paraphenylenediamine exposure.

Fig. 36.50 Albinism.

Fig. 36.51 Hermansky-Pudlak syndrome.

Fig. 36.52 Hermansky-Pudlak syndrome.

Fig. 36.53 Heterochromia.

Fig. 36.54 Piebaldism.

Fig. 36.55 Piebaldism.

Fig. 36.56 Piebaldism.

Fig. 36.57 Piebaldism.

Fig. 36.58 Piebaldism.

INDEX

Page numbers followed by "*f*" indicate figures.

A

"ABCDs" of melanoma, 463
Acanthoma, 438*f*
Acanthosis
  in breast skin, 3*f*
  neoplasms with, 437
Acanthosis nigricans, 347*f*–348*f*
  with malignancy, 348*f*
Acid burn, 65*f*
Acne, 169–183
  with 21-hydroxylase deficiency, 174*f*
  childhood, 170*f*
  cosmetica, 176*f*
  cyst with scarring, 173*f*
  excoriée, 176*f*
  fulminans, 174*f*–175*f*
  hirsutism and, 527*f*
    with Cushing disease, 174*f*
  with hyperpigmentation, 173*f*
  keloidalis, 178*f*
  keloids resulting from, 175*f*
  mechanica, 176*f*
  mild to moderate, 171*f*–172*f*
  moderate to severe, 172*f*
  neonatal, 169*f*
  pomade, 176*f*
  preadolescent, 171*f*
  scarring, 175*f*
  severe, 172*f*–173*f*
  severe infantile, 170*f*
  severe truncal, 173*f*
    with hyperpigmentation, 173*f*
  steroid, 177*f*
Acquired dyskeratotic leukoplakia, 552*f*
Acquired partial lipodystrophy, 336*f*–337*f*
Acral persistent papular mucinosis, 121*f*
Acrodermatitis chronica atrophicans, 202*f*
Acrodermatitis continua, 137*f*
Acrodermatitis enteropathica, 326*f*–327*f*
Acrokeratoelastoidosis, 148*f*
Acrokeratosis verruciformis of Hopf, 395*f*
Acromegaly, 339*f*–340*f*
Acropachy, thyroid, 346*f*
Acrospiroma, 453*f*
Actinic cheilitis, 543*f*
Actinic dermatitis, chronic, 35*f*
Actinic granuloma, 485*f*
Actinic prurigo, 34*f*
Actinomycosis, 195*f*
Acute generalized exanthematous pustulosis, 76*f*–77*f*
Acute hemorrhagic edema, of infancy, 570*f*–571*f*
Acute myelogenous leukemia, 17*f*
Acute necrotizing ulcerative gingivostomatitis, 557*f*
Acute paronychia, 187*f*
Acute shoe dermatitis, 68*f*

Acute systemic lupus erythematosus, 106*f*–107*f*
Acute urticaria, 18*f*
AD. *see* Atopic dermatitis (AD).
Adenomas, sebaceous, of Muir Torre syndrome, 450*f*
Adrenogenital syndrome, 342*f*–343*f*
Adult linear IgA disease, 320*f*
Ainhum, 421*f*
Alagille disease, lichen simplex chronicus in, 42*f*
Alagille syndrome, palmar striae in, 373*f*
Albinism, 592*f*
Alkaptonuria, 376*f*–377*f*
Allergic contact cheilitis, to topical steroids, 543*f*
Allergic shiners, 53
Alopecia
  androgenetic
    in man, 519*f*
    in woman, 519*f*
  central centrifugal cicatricial, 521*f*–522*f*
  congenital triangular, 520*f*
  frontal fibrosing, 521*f*
  in sarcoidosis, 492*f*
  scarring, secondary to discoid lupus erythematosus, 521*f*
  secondary syphilis, 258*f*
  in systemic lupus erythematosus, 107*f*
  traction, 522*f*–523*f*
Alopecia areata, 26*f*, 517*f*
  of beard, 518*f*
  in Down syndrome patient, 518*f*
  nails of patient with, 519*f*
  ophiasis type of, 518*f*
  recurrent, 518*f*
Alopecia mucinosa, 520*f*
  associated with mycosis fungoides, 507*f*
Alopecia neoplastica, from metastatic breast cancer, 432*f*, 523*f*
Alopecia universalis, 518*f*
Amalgam tattoo, 555*f*
Amantadine, livedo reticularis caused by, 562*f*
Amiodarone hyperpigmentation, 79*f*
Amyloidosis, 361, 361*f*–363*f*
  dyschromic, 365*f*
  lichen, 363*f*–364*f*
  macroglossia in, 362*f*
  macular, 363*f*
  nodular, 364*f*–365*f*
Androgenetic alopecia
  in man, 519*f*
  in woman, 519*f*
Anemia, smooth tongue in, 328*f*
Anergic leishmaniasis, 293*f*–294*f*
Anetoderma, 358*f*
Angioedema, 99*f*
Angioimmunoblastic T-cell lymphoma, 516*f*
Angiokeratoma
  circumscriptum, 411*f*
  of Fordyce, 411*f*–412*f*
  of Mibelli, 411*f*

Angiokeratoma corporis diffusum. *see* Fabry disease.
Angiolymphoid hyperplasia, with eosinophilia, 412*f*
Angiomas
  cherry, 415*f*
  circumscriptum, 411*f*
  serpiginosum, 413*f*
  spider, 410*f*
  tufted, 416*f*
Angiomatosis, diffuse dermal, 417*f*
Angiosarcoma, 418*f*–419*f*
Angular artery and vein, 13*f*
Angular cheilitis, 203, 544*f*
  in iron deficiency, 328*f*
Ankyloblepharon-ectodermal dysplasia-clefting, 398*f*
Annular atrophic panniculitis, 337*f*
Annular elastolytic granuloma, 484*f*–485*f*
Annular genital sarcoid, 488*f*
Annular lichen planus, 160*f*
Annular psoriasis, 133*f*
Annular sarcoidosis, 488*f*
Annulus migrans, 548*f*
Anonychia, 532*f*
Anthrax, with severe edema, 193*f*
Antibiotic allergy, leg ulcer with contact dermatitis due to, 72*f*
Antiphospholipid antibodies, in systemic lupus erythematosus, 109*f*
Apert syndrome, 403*f*
Aphthous stomatitis, 558*f*
Aplasia cutis congenita, 399*f*
Apocrine glands, in axillary skin, 3*f*
Aquagenic wrinkling, 150*f*
Aromatherapy, hand dermatitis due to, 71*f*
Arsenic, pigmentary changes from, 588*f*
Arterial ulceration, 581*f*
Arteriosclerosis obliterans, 577*f*
Arteriovenous fistula, 409*f*
Arteriovenous malformation syndrome, RASA1-associated, capillary malformation due to, 408*f*
Arteritis, temporal, 576*f*
Ascher syndrome, blepharochalasis in, 357*f*
Aspergillus infection, 203, 226*f*–227*f*
Asymmetric periflexural exanthem, of childhood, 278*f*–279*f*
Ataxia telangiectasia, 60*f*, 386*f*
Atopic dermatitis (AD), 53–64, 53*f*–56*f*
  chronic, 54*f*–55*f*
    with hyperpigmentation, 55*f*
  with Dennie-Morgan lines, 56*f*
  erythroderma from, 56*f*, 151*f*
  with excoriations, 54*f*
  hyperlinear palms in patient with, 57*f*
  lichenification, 55*f*
  papular, 56*f*
  with secondary infection, 54*f*–55*f*
Atrichia, with papular lesions, 523*f*
Atrophic lichen planus, 160*f*

Atrophic tongue, in vitamin B deficiencies, 323*f*
Atrophoderma, 24*f*
   of Pasini and Pierini, 113*f*
Atrophy blanche, 563*f*
Atypical fibroxanthoma, 425*f*
Atypical mycobacterial infections, 229
Auricular nerve, 14*f*
Auriculotemporal nerve, 10*f*
Autoinoculation vaccinia, 20*f*
Autosomal-recessive congenital ichthyosis with collodion membrane, 389*f*
   due to transglutaminase gene mutation with collodion membrane, 390*f*
   lamellar phenotype, 390*f*
Axillary freckling neurofibromatosis, 15*f*
Axillary granular parakeratosis, 348*f*
Axillary skin, 3*f*

B

Bacillary angiomatosis, 199*f*
Bacterial infections, 185–202
Bandage, contact allergy to adhesive in, 70*f*
Bart syndrome, 387*f*
Basal cell cancer, chronic radiodermatitis with, 35*f*
Basal cell carcinoma, 443*f*–444*f*
   aggressive, 444*f*
   large, 444*f*
   morpheaform, 444*f*
   nevus sebaceous with, 450*f*
   pigmented, 444*f*
   in radiation site, 445*f*
   skin tag-like, basal cell nevus syndrome with, 445*f*
   superficial, 443*f*
   tumor, 18*f*
   ulcer, 22*f*–23*f*
Basal cell nevus syndrome, 445*f*
Bazex syndrome, 434*f*
B-cell lymphoma, 513*f*
   leg type, 514*f*
Beau lines, 533*f*
Becker nevus, 466*f*–467*f*
Bedbug bites, 300*f*
Bee sting, 302*f*
Behçet disease, 559*f*
Bejel, 251–261, 260*f*
Benign follicular mucinosis, 122*f*–123*f*
Benzocaine, allergy to, 71*f*
Biliary cirrhosis
   palmar striae xanthoma in, 373*f*
   plane xanthoma in, 373*f*
   primary, tuberoeruptive xanthomas and, 372*f*
Birt-Hogg-Dubé syndrome, 458*f*
Bites, 291–307
   of bedbug, 300*f*
   of brown recluse spider, 307*f*
   of *Cheyletiella* mite, 306*f*
   of chigger, 306*f*
   of flea, 302*f*–303*f*
   of insect, 299*f*
   of Russell pit viper, 307*f*
   of snake, 307*f*
   of spider, 307*f*
   of tick, 303*f*
   of Triatome, 294*f*

Black dermatographism, 69*f*
Black hairy tongue, 549*f*
Black heel, 37*f*
Blastomycosis, North American, 220*f*–221*f*
Bleomycin flagellate hyperpigmentation, 81*f*
Blepharochalasis, in Ascher syndrome, 357*f*
Blistering and atrophy, in complex regional pain syndrome, 51*f*
Blistering dactylitis, 192*f*
Blisters, factitial, 49*f*
Blistik, contact cheilitis to, 72*f*
Bloom syndrome, 403*f*
Blue dye dermatitis, 68*f*
Blue rubber bleb syndrome, 408*f*
Botryomycosis, 188*f*
Boutonneuse fever, 201*f*
Bowen disease, 447*f*–448*f*
   of nail bed, 540*f*
Bowenoid papulosis, 284*f*
BRAF inhibitor-induced hand-foot reaction, 83*f*
Breast
   nevus on, 469*f*
   Paget disease of, 448*f*–449*f*
Breast cancer
   ductal, 431*f*
   inflammatory, 432*f*
   male, metastases, 432*f*
Breast skin, 3*f*
Brocq, pseudopelade of, 522*f*
Brooke-Spiegler syndrome, 456*f*
Brown pigments, in cutaneous eruption, 1
Brown recluse spider bite, 307*f*
Bruising, factitial, 49*f*
Brunsting-Perry pemphigoid, 318*f*
Buccinators muscle, parotid duct piercing of, 11*f*
Buerger disease, 576*f*–577*f*
Buffalo hump, 341*f*
Bulb, hair, 5*f*–6*f*
Bulimia, vomiting with, enamel erosion secondary to, 47*f*
Bullous diabetic dermatosis, 376*f*
Bullous impetigo, 189*f*
Bullous mastocytosis, 426*f*
Bullous pemphigoid, 315*f*
   erosion, 22*f*
   vesicles and bullae, 19*f*
Bullous systemic lupus erythematosus, 107*f*–108*f*
Bullous tinea pedis, 208*f*
Burn scar, 28*f*
Burns
   acid, 65*f*
   cement, 65*f*
   dig, from acid solution, 66*f*
   pesticide, 66*f*
   senna, 66*f*
Buruli ulcer, 235*f*
Buschke-Lowenstein tumor, 284*f*
Buschke-Ollendorff syndrome, 422*f*

C

Calabar swelling, 298*f*
Calcinosis cutis, 361, 369*f*
Calciphylaxis, 368*f*, 564*f*
Candidal infections, 203

Candidal sepsis, 214*f*–215*f*
Candidiasis, 210*f*–213*f*
   chronic, common variable immunodeficiency with, 61*f*
   chronic mucocutaneous, 213*f*–214*f*
   thrush in, 210*f*
   congenital, 203, 212*f*
   oral, 210*f*
Capillary, in papillary dermis, 5*f*
Capillary malformation (port-wine stain), 407*f*
   with Sturge-Weber syndrome, 407*f*
Carbon stain, in gunshot wound, 39*f*
Carcinoid syndrome, 435*f*
Carcinoma
   adnexal, microcystic, 455*f*
   basal cell, 443*f*–444*f*
      aggressive, 444*f*
      large, 444*f*
      morpheaform, 444*f*
      nevus sebaceous with, 450*f*
      pigmented, 444*f*
      in radiation site, 445*f*
      skin tag-like, basal cell nevus syndrome with, 445*f*
      superficial, 443*f*
      tumor, 18*f*
      ulcer, 22*f*–23*f*
   Merkel cell, 449*f*
   sebaceous, 450*f*
   squamous cell, 446*f*
      Bowen disease with, 447*f*
   verrucous, 447*f*
Carcinoma erysipeloides, 432*f*
Carney syndrome, 465*f*, 588*f*
Carotenemia, 330*f*
Cartilage, in early spine formation, 1*f*
Cat scratch disease, 199*f*
Catastrophic antiphospholipid antibody syndrome, 566*f*
Cavernous venous malformation, 408*f*
CD30+ anaplastic T-cell lymphoma, 511*f*
Cellulitis, 180*f*, 191*f*
Cement burns, 65*f*
Central centrifugal cicatricial alopecia, 521*f*–522*f*
Cephalic histiocytosis, benign, 494*f*, 497*f*
Cerebrotendinous xanthomas, 373*f*
Ceruminous glands, in ear canal, 2*f*
Chagas disease, Romana sign in, 294*f*
Chancroid, 197*f*
Cheilitis
   actinic, 543*f*
   allergic contact, to topical steroids, 543*f*
   angular, 203, 544*f*
   granulomatous, 547*f*
   plasma cell, 544*f*
   secondary to lip licking, 543*f*
Cheilitis glandularis, 544*f*
Chemotherapy
   toxic erythema of, 82*f*
   transverse nail bands secondary to, 537*f*
Chemotherapy-induced transverse nail hyperpigmentation, 80*f*
Cherry angiomas, and costal fringe telangiectases, 415*f*
Cheyletiella mite bites, 306*f*
Chigger bites, 306*f*
Chikungunya fever, 280*f*
Chilblain systemic lupus erythematosus, 107*f*

Childhood, asymmetric periflexural exanthem in, 278f–279f
Childhood acne, 170f
Childhood linear IgA disease, 321f
Childhood pityriasis rubra pilaris, 144f
Chloracne, 177f
Chloroquine hyperpigmentation, 81f, 554f
Chlorpromazine hyperpigmentation, 79f, 554f
Cholesterol emboli, 563f
Cholinergic urticaria, 97f–98f
Chondrodermatitis nodularis chronica helices, 423f
Chromomycosis, 223f
Chronic blistering dermatoses, 309–322
Chronic hand dermatitis, from cement, 21f
Chronic mucocutaneous candidiasis, 213f–214f
Chronic shoe dermatitis, 68f
Chronic solar damage, 32f
Chrysiasis, 79f
Cicatricial pemphigoid, 317f–318f
Cigarette burn, factitial, 48f
Circumscribed juvenile pityriasis rubra pilaris, 145f
Cirrhosis, primary biliary, hyperpigmentation in, 42f
Clonidine patch allergy, 71f
Closed comedones, 171f
Clostridial ulcer, 194f
Clothing contact dermatitis, 68f
CLOVE syndrome, 438f
Clubbing, 531f
Coccidioidomycosis, 203, 218f–219f
Cockayne syndrome, 402f
Cockayne-xeroderma pigmentosum syndrome, 402f
Coin rubbing, purpura from, 567f
Cold panniculitis, 335f–336f
Cold urticaria, 19f, 97f
Collagenous and elastic marginal plaques, of hands, 148f
Colloid milium, 32f
Comedones
  closed, 171f
  open, 170f–171f
Complex regional pain syndrome, 50f–51f
Compulsive finger biting, 46f
Condyloma lata, 257f
Condylomata acuminata, 283f
Confluent and reticulated papillomatosis, 140f
Congenital anomalies, genodermatoses and, 379–404
Congenital candidiasis, 203, 212f
Congenital hemidysplasia, with ichthyosiform erythroderma and limb defects syndrome, 392f
Congenital hypothyroidism, 343f
Congenital ichthyosiform erythroderma, 21f
Congenital onychodysplasia, of index finger, 532f
Congenital syphilis, 259f
  with Hutchinson teeth, 259f
  with mulberry molar, 259f
  with scars from rhagades, 260f
Congenital triangular alopecia, 520f
Conjunctiva, lipodermoid of, Schimmelpenning syndrome with, 438f

Conjunctival erythema, reactive arthritis with, 135f
Connective tissue disease, 101–118
Connective tissue nevus, 421f–422f
Conradi-Hunermann syndrome, 380f
Contact allergy
  to adhesive in bandage, 70f
  to steroids, 72f
Contact cheilitis, to Blistex, 72f
Contact dermatitis, 65–85
  to eye drops, 72f
  leg ulcer with, 72f
Contact urticaria, to surgical gloves, 72f
Coral granuloma, 296f
Costal fringe telangiectases, cherry angiomas and, 415f
Cotton granuloma, 38f
Cough-induced purpura, 567f
Cowden syndrome, 457f
Coxsackie A6 hand-foot-and-mouth disease, 277f
Cradle cap, 126f
Crohn disease, cutaneous, 545f–546f
Crusted scabies, in HIV-infected patient, 306f
Cryoglobulinemic vasculitis, 565f, 571f–572f
Cryopyrin-associated periodic fever syndrome
  with atypical pernio-like lesion, 96f
  with Muckle-Wells syndrome, 96f
Cryptococcal infection, 220f
  in an HIV-infected patient, 220f
Cuboidal periderm, in early fetal life, 1f
Culprit swim goggles, 70f
Curth-Macklin with keratin 1 mutation, ichthyosis hystrix of, 147f
Cushing disease, 340f
  hypertrichosis in, 341f
  skin thinning and ecchymoses in, 341f
Cutaneous collagenous vasculopathy, 579f
Cutaneous Crohn disease, 545f–546f
Cutaneous dental sinus, 550f
Cutaneous diphtheria, 193f
Cutaneous larva migrans, 291, 297f
Cutaneous mucin deposition, 119
Cutaneous *Mycobacterium avium-intracellulare* infection, 237f
Cutaneous *Mycobacterium kansasii* infection, 237f
Cutaneous vascular diseases, 561–581
Cutis laxa, 357f
Cutis marmorata telangiectatica congenita, 406f
Cutis rhomboidalis nuchae, 31f
Cutis verticis gyrata, 399f
Cylindroma, 454f
Cysts
  acne, with scarring, 173f
  dermoid, 460f
  epidermal, 437–462
  epidermal inclusion, 459f
  eruptive vellus hair, 461f
  labial, 459f
  median raphae, 462f
  pilar, 460f
  pilonidal, 460f
  scrotal, 459f
  thyroglossal duct, 462f
Cytomegaloviral infection, in newborn, 271f
Cytomegaloviral ulcer, in HIV-infected patient, 272f

D

Darier disease, 16f, 394f–395f
  erythronychia in, 536f
  of nail, 531f
Decubitus ulcer, 37f
Deep lymphatic malformation, 410f
Degos disease, 576f
Delayed pressure urticaria, 98f
Delusions of parasitosis, 47f
Demodex mites, in facial skin, 2f
Dengue, 280f
Dennie-Morgan lines, atopic dermatitis with, 56f
Dental impression material allergy, stomatitis due to, 70f
Depigmentation, secondary to paraphenylenediamine exposure, 592f
Dermal and subcutaneous tumors, 405–435
Dermal dendrocyte hamartoma, 424f
Dermal duct tumor, 453f
Dermal fibrous tissue, abnormalities of, 351–359
Dermatitis
  actinic, chronic, 35f
  acute shoe, 68f
  atopic, 53–64, 53f–56f
    chronic, 54f–55f
    with Dennie-Morgan lines, 56f
    erythroderma from, 56f
    with excoriations, 54f
    hyperlinear palms in, 57f
    with hyperpigmentation, chronic, 55f
    lichenification, 55f
    papular, 56f
    with secondary infection, 54f–55f
  blue dye, 68f
  chronic hand, from cement, 21f
  chronic shoe, 68f
  clothing contact, 68f
  contact, 65–85
    to eye drops, 72f
    leg ulcer with, 72f
  earbud, 70f
  eyelid, 71f
  factitial, 48f
  finger, from primrose allergy, 58f
  fire coral, 295f
  hair dye, 71f
  hand, 71f
    with secondary infection, 58f
  herpetiformis, 309, 319f–320f
  irritant, from kerosene, 66f
  irritant diaper, 59f
  jellyfish, 295f
  Katayama fever-associated, 296f
  nickel, 69f
  oral lichenoid, 70f
  Paederus, 302f
  phytophotodermatitis, 33f
  poison ivy, 65, 67f
  Portuguese man of war, 295f
  radiodermatitis, chronic, 35f
  rubber, 70f
  sea wasp, 295f
  seaweed, 296f
  stasis, 580f–581f

Dermatitis (Continued)
　　tea tree oil, 67f
　　vulvar, 71f
Dermatofibroma, 405, 423f–424f
　　multiple, 424f
　　sarcoma protuberans, 17f, 424f–425f
Dermatographism, 87, 98f–99f
　　white, 56f
Dermatology, field of, 517
Dermatomyositis (DM), 111f
　　with calcification, 112f
　　Gottron's papules, 110f
　　heliotrope, 109f
　　mechanic's hands, 111f
　　Samitz sign, 110f
　　shawl sign, 111f
　　with ulceration, 112f
Dermatopathia pigmentosa reticularis, 586f
Dermatophyte infections, 203
Dermatophytoma, 209f
Dermatoses, resulting from physical factors, 27–39, 33f
Dermatosis papulosa nigra, 440f
Dermoscopy, 463
Desmosome, 6f
Diabetic dermopathy, 376f
Diabetic gangrene, 376f
Diapers, blue dye dermatitis and, 68f
Diffuse hyperkeratosis, of the palms, 147f
Diffuse leprosy of Lucio, 246f
Digital sarcoidosis, 490f
Digital ulcers, Raynaud phenomenon with, 561f
Digitate parapsoriasis, 139f
Dilated follicular orifices, 119
Discoid lupus erythematosus, 23f, 101f–103f
　　generalized, 103f
　　of scalp, 520f
　　scarring alopecia secondary to, 521f
Disseminated herpes simplex infection, 267f
Disseminated sporotrichosis, 223f
Disseminated vaccinia, 274f
DM. see Dermatomyositis (DM).
DOCK8 immunodeficiency, warts in, 61f–62f
Dominant dystrophic epidermolysis bullosa, 387f
Doxorubicin hyperpigmentation, 79f–80f
Doxycycline, photoonycholysis secondary to, 33f
Drip burn, from acid solution, 66f
Drug eruptions, 16f, 65–85, 73f
　　in leukemic patient, 73f
Drug-induced antineutrophil cytoplasmic antibody-positive vasculitis, 574f
Dryness, secondary to compulsive hand washing, 46f
Ductal breast cancer, 431f
Dupuytren contracture, 420f
Dyschromatosis symmetrica hereditaria, 584f–585f
Dyschromatosis universalis hereditaria, 586f–587f
Dyschromic amyloidosis, 365f
Dyshidrosis, 19f
Dyskeratomas, warty, 439f
Dyskeratosis congenita, 396f–397f
Dyspigmentation, in systemic sclerosis, 115f
Dystrophic calcinosis cutis, 367f

E

Ear
　　anatomy of, 10f
　　juvenile spring eruption of, 34f
　　skin of, 2f
Ear canal, skin of, 2f
Ear eczema, 58f
Early follicular hyperkeratosis, pityriasis rubra pilaris with, 142f
Early scleromyxedema, 119f
Earphone dermatitis, 70f
Earrings, nickel dermatitis with, 69f
Eccrine acrospiroma, 453f
Eccrine carcinoma, 455f
Eccrine glands, in volar skin, 5f
Eccrine porocarcinoma, 454f
Eccrine poroma, 452f–453f
Eccrine spiradenoma, 453f
Ecthyma, 190f
Ecthyma gangrenosum, 195f–196f
Ectrodactyly ectodermal dysplasia-clefting, 398f
Eczema, 53–64
　　ear, 58f
　　eyelid, 58f
　　herpeticum, 57f, 267f
　　nipple, in atopic child, 58f
　　nummular, 59f
　　in Wiskott-Aldrich syndrome, 60f
　　xerotic, 59f
Edema
　　acute hemorrhagic, of infancy, 570f–571f
　　rounded scars and, from skin popping, 23f
EDS. see Ehlers-Danlos syndrome (EDS).
Ehlers-Danlos syndrome (EDS), 354f–357f
Elastic tissue, abnormalities of, 351–359
Elastosis, solar, of the forehead, 32f
Elastosis perforans serpiginosa, 351f, 354f
Elastotic striae, 359f
Electrical burn, from biting electrical cord, 28f
Emphysema, subcutaneous, 37f
Enamel erosion secondary to vomiting with bulimia, 47f
Encephalocele, 428f–429f
Endocrine diseases, 339–349
Endometriosis, cutaneous, 431f
Eosinophil, 7f
Eosinophilia, phenytoin-induced drug reaction with, 73f–74f
Eosinophilic annular erythema, 92f
Eosinophilic fasciitis, 116f
Eosinophilic folliculitis, in HIV-infected patient, 289f
Eosinophilic granulomatosis with polyangiitis, 575f
Epidemic typhus, 200f
Epidermal growth factor inhibitor-induced acneiform reaction, 83f
Epidermal growth factor inhibitor-induced paronychia, 83f
Epidermodysplasia verruciformis, in HIV-infected patient, 285f
Epidermolysis bullosa
　　dominant dystrophic, 387f
　　junctional, 386f
　　recessive dystrophic, 387f
Epidermolysis bullosa acquisita, 318f–319f
Epidermolysis bullosa simplex, 19f
　　generalized, 386f
　　localized, 386f
Epidermolytic ichthyosis, 390f–391f
Epithelioid sarcoma, 425f
Epulis, 556f
Erb point, 13f
Erosio interdigitalis blastomycetica, 213f
Erosions, factitial, 49f
Erosive lichen planus, 159f
Erosive pustular dermatitis, of scalp, 522f
Eruptive histiocytomas, generalized, 494f
Eruptive xanthomas, 16f, 369f–370f
Erysipelas, 190f–191f
Erysipeloid, 193f
Erythema, 87–99
Erythema ab igne, 25f, 29f
Erythema annulare centrifugum, 91f
Erythema dyschromicum perstans, 162f–163f
Erythema elevatum diutinum, 572f
Erythema gyratum repens, 91f
Erythema induratum, 229, 233f, 331, 333f
Erythema infectiosum, 279f
Erythema marginatum, 192f–193f
Erythema migrans, 201f–202f
Erythema multiforme, 88f–89f
　　recurrent oral, 90f–91f
Erythema nodosum, 18f, 331f–333f
Erythema nodosum leprosum, 239
Erythema nodosum-like sarcoidosis, 491f
Erythema toxicum neonatorum, 88f
Erythematotelangiectatic rosacea, 180f
Erythrasma, 193f–194f
Erythroderma, 125–138
　　from atopic dermatitis, 56f, 151f
Erythrodermic bullous pemphigoid, 316f
Erythrodermic psoriasis, 134f
Erythrodermic sarcoidosis, 492f
Erythrokeratoderma variabilis, 393f
Erythromelalgia, 561f–562f
Erythronychia, in Darier disease, 536f
Erythroplasia of Queyrat, 448f
Erythropoietic protoporphyria, 366f–367f
Excoriation, 41
　　atopic dermatitis with, 54f
　　Hodgkin disease, secondary to pruritus of, 41f
　　prurigo nodularis with, 46f
　　psychogenic, 47f
Exercise-induced urticaria, 97f
Exogenous nail staining, 538f
Exogenous ochronosis, 377f
Exophthalmos, 346f
Extensive warts, 282f–283f
External carotid artery, 13f
External jugular vein, 13f–14f
Extremities, skin tension lines in, 9f
Eyelid, anatomy of, 4f
Eyelid dermatitis, 71f
Eyelid eczema, 58f
Eyelid lichen planus, 161f

F

Fabry disease, 375f
Face, arterial and venous supply of, 13f
Facial artery and vein, 13f–14f
Facial dermatitis, granulomatous, 182f–183f
Facial expression, muscles of, 11f

Index

Facial nerve, anatomy of, 11f
Facial skin, 2f
    innervation of, 12f
    major anatomic landmarks in, 10f
Factitial blisters, 49f
Factitial bruising, 49f
Factitial dermatitis, 48f
Factitial erosions, 49f
Factitial lacerations, 49f
Factitial scarring, 49f
Factitial ulcers, 48f-49f
Fasciitis, 191f-192f
    in graft-*versus*-host disease, 64f
Fat, subcutaneous, lobules of, 5f
Favre-Racouchot syndrome, 31f
Fibrokeratoma, acquired digital, 422f
Fibroma
    sclerotic, 458f
    secondary to chronic tongue biting, 47f
Fibrosis, chronic radiodermatitis with, 35f
Fibrous papule, of nose, 422f
Filariasis, 297f-298f
Finger biting, compulsive, 46f
Finger dermatitis, from primrose allergy, 58f
Fire ant stings, 302f
Fire coral cuts, 36f
Fire coral dermatitis, 295f
Fissured tongue, 548f
Fixed cutaneous sporotrichosis, 222f
Fixed drug reaction, 75f-76f
Flag sign, 524f
Flea bites, 302f-303f
Flegel disease, 440f
Fluoroscopy-induced radiodermatitis, 36f
Flushing, 87f
Focal acral hyperkeratosis, 148f-149f
Focal cutaneous mucinosis, 124f
Fogo selvagem, 21f, 313f
Follicular accentuation, 1
Follicular iododerma, 84f
Follicular mucinosis, 119
    associated with mycosis fungoides, 123f
Folliculitis, 1
    Pityrosporum, 218f
    staphylococcal, 20f
Folliculitis decalvans, 522f
Foot, immersion, tropical, 30f
Fordyce spots, 547f
Forehead, medial, 12f
Forschheimer spots, in rubella, 278f
Fox-Fordyce disease, 529f
    with xanthomatous change, 529f
Frontal fibrosing alopecia, 161f, 521f
Frostbite, 30f
Fungal infections, 203
Fungi, diseases resulting from, 203-227
Fusarium infection, 203, 226f

G

GA. *see* Granuloma annulare (GA).
Galli-Galli disease, 585f
Gamma-delta T-cell lymphoma, 512f
Generalized discoid lupus erythematosus, 103f
Generalized essential telangiectasia, 579f
Generalized *Mycobacterium avium-intracellulare* infection, 237f
Genital sarcoidosis, 488f
Genital warts, 284f

Genodermatoses, 379-404
Geographic tongue, 548f
Gianotti-Crosti syndrome, 263, 273f
Giant cell tumor, of tendon sheath, 421f
Giant molluscum contagiosum, 275f-276f
Glandular rosacea, 181f
    with rhinophyma, 181f
Glioma, nasal, 428f
Globi, 239
Glomangioma, 416f-417f
Glucagonoma, 433f-434f
Glucocorticoid excess, striae in, 341f
Gnathostomiasis, 297f
Gold, oral lichenoid dermatitis due to, 70f
Goltz syndrome, 399f-400f
Gonococcal infection, 198f
Gonococcemia, 198f
Gout, 377f-378f
Graft-*versus*-host disease
    acute, 62f-63f
    chronic, 63f-64f
    fasciitis in, 64f
    grade 2, acute, 62f
    grade 4, acute, 62f
    lichenoid, 63f
    sclerodermoid type, chronic, 63f-64f
Graham-Little-Piccardi syndrome, 162f
Gram-negative folliculitis, 177f-178f
Gram-negative toe web infection, 196f
Granular cell tumor, 405, 427f
    multiple, 427f
Granulation tissue, on isotretinoin, 176f
Granulocyte colony stimulating factor reaction, 84f
Granuloma, pyogenic, 18f, 412f-413f, 556f
Granuloma annulare (GA), 24f, 479, 479f-483f
    deep, 483f
    disseminated, 482f-483f
    facial, 484f
    perforating, 483f
    subcutaneous, 484f
Granuloma faciale, 573f
Granuloma inguinale, 197f-198f
Granulomatosis with polyangiitis, 574f-575f
Granulomatous cheilitis, 547f
Granulomatous facial dermatitis, 182f-183f
Granulomatous lesion, in ataxia telangiectasia, 61f
Granulomatous slack skin, 509f
Greater auricular nerve enlargement, in leprosy, 241f
Green nail, 538f
    from *Pseudomonas* infection, 26f
Guttate psoriasis, 132f

H

Haemophilus influenzae cellulitis, 197f
Hailey-Hailey disease, 20f, 387f-388f
Hair
    anatomy of, 5f-6f
    diseases of, 517
    progressive kinking of, 526f
Hair collar sign, 399f
Hair dye dermatitis, 71f

Hair follicles, in scalp skin, 3f
Hair granuloma, in barber, 38f
Hairy leukoplakia, 271f
Half-and-half nails, 533f
Hamartoma
    basiloid follicular, 459f
    smooth muscle, 431f
Hand, neuropathic ulcer of, 51f
Hand dermatitis, 71f
    with secondary infection, 58f
Hand washing, compulsive, dryness secondary to, 46f
Hand-foot-and-mouth disease, 276f-277f
Hansen disease, 239-250
Hard corn, 36f
Harlequin fetus, 390f
Headlight sign, 53
Heel, black, 37f
Heel stick calcinosis, 368f
Hemangioma
    infantile, 413f-414f
        involuting, 414f-415f
        with ulceration, 414f
    spindle cell, 417f
    targetoid hemosiderotic, 415f
Hemangiomatosis, diffuse neonatal, 415f
Henoch-Schönlein purpura, 570f
Hepatic cholestasis, xanthomas of the palmar crease in, 42f
Hermansky-Pudlak syndrome, 592f
Herpangina, 276f
Herpes genitalis, 266f
Herpes gladiatorum, 265f
Herpes simplex infection, 25f
    disseminated, 267f
    intrauterine, 267f
    primary, 263f-264f
    recurrent, 264f-265f
    ulcerative, 268f
Herpes zoster, 269f-271f
Herpetic sycosis, 265f
Herpetic whitlow, 265f
Heterochromia, 592f
Hidradenitis suppurativa, 169, 178f-180f
Hidradenoma, nodular, 453f
Hidrocystoma, 452f
Hidrotic ectodermal dysplasia, 398f
Hirsutism, acne and, 527f
Histiocytoid leprosy, 246f
Histiocytoid Sweet syndrome, 94f
Histiocytosis
    cephalic, 494f, 497f
    Langerhans cell. *see* Langerhans cell histiocytosis (LCH).
    malignant, 514f
    progressive nodular, 495f
Histoplasmosis, 203, 219f
HIV-infected patient
    acquired ichthyosis in, 289f
    chronic herpes simplex in, 286f
    condylomata acuminatum in, 287f
    crusted scabies in, 288f, 306f
    cryptococcal infection in, 220f
    cytomegaloviral ulcer in, 272f
    eosinophilic folliculitis in, 289f
    epidermodysplasia verruciformis in, 285f, 287f
    generalized *Mycobacterium avium-intracellulare* infection in, 237f
    hair straightening in, 288f

HIV-infected patient (Continued)
  herpes simplex and seborrheic dermatitis in, 286f
  herpes zoster in, 271f, 287f
  Kaposi sarcoma in, 272f, 288f
  long eyelashes in, 289f
  molluscum contagiosum in, 287f
  oral hairy leukoplakia in, 288f
  proximal white onychomycosis in, 286f
  reactive arthritis in, 289f
  secondary syphilis in, 255f
  sulfa allergy in, 75f
  thrush in, 286f
  ulcerative herpes simplex in, 268f, 287f
Hodgkin disease, excoriations secondary to pruritus of, 41f
Homozygous familial hypercholesterolemia, xanthomas in, 17f
Homozygous protein C deficiency, 566f
Horn, cutaneous, 441f
Hot oil burn, 28f
Hot tub folliculitis, 196f–197f
Hot water bottle injury, 27f
Hot water burn, 27f
HTLV-1 dermatosis, 285f
Hunter syndrome, 377f
Hutchinson teeth, congenital syphilis with, 259f
Hydroa vacciniforme, 34f
Hydroa vacciniforme-like natural killer T-cell lymphoma, 512f–513f
Hypercholesterolemia
  homozygous familial, xanthomas in, 17f
  with intertriginous xanthomas, 371f–372f
Hypereosinophilic syndrome, 516f
Hyperkeratosis
  diffuse, 147f
  focal acral, 148f–149f
  neoplasms with, 437
  in psoriatic nails, 530f
  spiny, 146f
  in volar skin, 4f
Hyperkeratotic diseases, 139–151
Hyperlinear palms, in atopic dermatitis, 57f
Hyperpigmentation
  in Addison disease, 341f–342f
  chronic atopic dermatitis with, 55f
  familial progressive, 587f
  of hand and cheek after phytophotodermatitis, 33f
  in primary biliary cirrhosis, 42f
  seborrheic dermatitis with, 126f
Hyperplasia, sebaceous, 450f
Hypersensitivity, piroxicam, 19f
Hypertrichosis
  in Cushing disease, 341f
  localized, 527f
  from minoxidil, 527f
Hypertrichosis cubiti, 527f
Hypertrophic lichen planus, 156f–157f
Hypertrophic lupus erythematosus, 17f, 103f
Hypertrophic osteoarthropathy, from lung cancer, 434f
Hypohidrotic X-linked ectodermal dysplasia, 397f–398f
Hypopigmentation
  after intralesional steroid injection, 85f
  familial progressive, 587f
  overlying sarcoidosis, 490f
  seborrheic dermatitis with, 127f
Hypothyroidism, 344f

I

Ichthyosiform erythroderma, congenital, 21f
Ichthyosiform sarcoidosis, 491f–492f
Ichthyosis
  acquired
    in leprosy, 247f
    in myeloma patient, 434f
  autosomal-recessive congenital
    with collodion membrane, 389f–390f
    lamellar phenotype, 390f
  epidermolytic, 390f–391f
  vulgaris, 388f–389f
    with hyperlinear palms, 389f
  X-linked, 21f, 389f
Ichthyosis hystrix, of Curth-Macklin with keratin 1 mutation, 147f
Id reaction, 59f, 204f
Idiopathic eruptive macular hyperpigmentation, with papillomatosis, 163f
IgA-mediated disease, 309
Immersion foot, tropical, 30f
Immune thrombocytopenic purpura, 564f–565f
Immunobullous dermatoses, 309
Impetigo, 20f, 188f
Incontinentia pigmenti
  early inflammatory phase, 379f
  with pigmentary lesions, 380f
  with verrucous lesions, 379f–380f
Indeterminate leprosy, 239f
Infantile acne, 170f
Infantile bullous pemphigoid, 316f
Infantile digital fibromas, 421f
Infantile hemangioma, 413f–414f
  involuting, 414f–415f
  with ulceration, 414f
Infantile psoriasis, 131f–132f
Infected human bite, 199f
Infections
  Aspergillus, 226f–227f
  atypical mycobacterial, 229
  bacterial, 185–202
  candidal, 203
  cryptococcal, 220f
    in HIV-infected patient, 220f
  dermatophyte, 203
  fungal, 203
  Fusarium, 226f
  gonococcal, 198f
  Gram-negative toe web, 196f
  mold, 203
  perianal streptococcal, 192f
  pseudomonal, green nail secondary to, 196f
  Rhizopus, 226f
  Vibrio vulnificus, 199f
Inferior labial artery, 13f–14f
Inflammatory bowel disease (IBD), mucosal diseases in, 543
Inflammatory breast cancer, 432f
Infraorbital crease, 10f
Infraorbital foramen, and related structures, 12f
Infundibulofolliculitis, disseminate and recurrent, 528f
Infundibulum, follicular, tumor of, 459f
Ink spot lentigo, 464f
Inoculation tuberculosis, primary, 229f

Insect bite, 299f
Insulin lipohypertrophy, 338f
Interdigital tinea, 207f
Internal jugular vein, 13f
Intertriginous xanthomas, hypercholesterolemia with, 371f–372f
Intertrigo, 194f
Intraepidermal neutrophilic IgA dermatosis, 314f
Intrauterine herpes simplex infection, 267f
Intravenous extravasation, with necrosis, 79f
Inverse psoriasis, 131f
Iron deficiency, angular cheilitis in, 328f
Irritant dermatitis, from kerosene, 66f
Irritant diaper dermatitis, 59f
Isomorphic (Koebner) phenomenon, 41
Isoniazid-induced pellagra-like reactions, 326f
Isotretinoin, granulation tissue on, 176f
Isotretinoin skin fragility, 22f
Itch, winter, 43f

J

Janeway spot, in staphylococcal endocarditis, 185f
Jaundice, 42f
Jellyfish dermatitis, 295f
Jessner lymphocytic infiltrate, of skin, 502f
Job's syndrome, 60f
Junctional epidermolysis bullosa, 386f
Juvenile spring eruption, of ears, 34f
Juvenile xanthogranulomas (JXG), 479, 493f
  large, 494f
  multiple, 494f
  plaque, 494f

K

Kaposi sarcoma, 26f
  in HIV-infected patient, 272f, 417f–418f
  secondary syphilis and, 255f
Kaposiform hemangioendothelioma, 416f
Kasabach-Merritt syndrome, 416f
Katayama fever-associated dermatitis, 296f
Kawasaki disease, 577f–578f
Keloid, 18f, 23f, 419f
  ulcerated, 419f
Keratinocytes, pale, 5f
Keratitis ichthyosis deafness syndrome, 392f
Keratoacanthoma, 442f
Keratoderma climactericum, 147f
Keratoderma of Vohwinkel, mutilating, 147f–148f
Keratolysis exfoliativa, 145f
Keratoses
  actinic, 441f
  arsenical, 440f
  lichenoid, benign, 440f
  seborrheic, 439f
  stucco, 440f
Keratosis follicularis spinulosa decalvans, 404f, 523f
Keratosis pilaris, 57f, 404f
Keratosis pilaris rubra faciei, 57f
Keratosis punctata, of palmar creases, 145f–146f
Kerion, 204f
Klippel-Trenaunay syndrome, 409f

Knuckle pads, 420f
Koebner phenomenon, 153, 155f
Koilonychia, 531f
  with trachyonychia, 531f
Koplik spots, 278f
Kwashiorkor, 328f–330f

L

Labiomental crease, 10f
Lacerations, factitial, 49f
Lamotrigine, toxic epidermal necrolysis to, 74f–75f
Langerhans cell, with Birbeck granules, 6f
Langerhans cell histiocytosis (LCH), 479, 497f–498f
  in adult, 499f
  congenital, 496f–497f
Larva migrans, cutaneous, 25f
Lateral nasal artery and vein, 13f
Laugier-Hunziker syndrome, 588f
LCH. see Langerhans cell histiocytosis (LCH).
Leiomyomas, 430f
  multiple, 430f
Leiomyosarcoma, 431f
Leishmaniasis
  anergic, 293f–294f
  mucocutaneous, 293f
  New World, 291f–293f
  Old World, 291f
  post-kala-azar dermal, 294f
Lentigines
  in LEOPARD syndrome, 465f
  solar, 464f
Lentiginosis
  generalized, 465f
  inherited patterned, 465f–466f
Lentigo maligna, 471f
Lentigo maligna melanoma, 472f
Lentigo simplex, 464f
LEOPARD syndrome, 381f
  lentigines in, 465f
Lepromatous leprosy, 244f–246f
  borderline, 243f–244f
Leprosy
  acquired ichthyosis in, 247f
  erythema nodosum leprosum reactional, 249f
  histiocytoid, 246f
  indeterminant, 239f
  lepromatous, 244f–246f
    borderline, 243f–244f
  of Lucio, 246f
  nerve enlargement in, 241f
    greater auricular, 241f
  neuropathic ulcer in, 247f
  secondary changes due to neurologic disease in, 247f
  tuberculoid, 239, 240f
    borderline, 241f–243f
    early, 239f
  type 1 reactional, 248f
  type 2 reactional, 249f
Leukemia, acute myelogenous, 17f
Leukemia cutis, 515f
Leukemic patient
  Aspergillus in, 226f–227f
  Fusarium infection in, 226f
Leukocytoclastic vasculitis, 569f

Leukonychia, 536f
  transverse, 536f
Leukoplakia, 550f
  acquired dyskeratotic, 552f
  cheilitis glandularis with, 544f
  oral hairy, 17f
Levamisole-induced vasculopathy, 575f–576f
Levator palpebrae superioris, 12f
Lichen amyloidosis, 363f–364f
Lichen aureus, 569f
Lichen nitidus, 153, 163f–165f
Lichen planopilaris, 161f, 521f
Lichen planus actinicus, 153, 162f
Lichen planus (LP), 24f, 153–168, 153f–157f, 159f–161f
  actinicus, 153, 162f
  after radiation therapy, 161f
  annular, 160f
  atrophic, 160f
  eyelid, 161f
  hypertrophic, 156f–157f
  oral, 158f
Lichen planus lupus erythematosus overlap, 104f
Lichen planus pigmentosus, 153, 162f
Lichen sclerosus, 153, 166f–168f
Lichen simplex chronicus, 24f, 44f–45f
  in Alagille disease, 42f
  with dyspigmentation and early nodule formation, 45f
  in pruritus ani, 43f
  of scrotum, 43f
  of vulva, 43f
Lichen striatus, 153, 165f–166f
Lichenification, 41, 53
  of atopic dermatitis, 55f
Lichenoid drug reaction, 81f
Lichenoid graft-*versus*-host disease, 63f
Lid margin, 4f
Linear epidermal nevus, 25f
Linear psoriasis, 132f
Lip lichen planus, 159f
Lip licking, chronic, 46f
Lipoatrophy, after steroid injection, 85f
Lipodermatosclerosis, 331, 333f–334f
Lipodystrophy, acquired partial, 336f–337f
Lipofuscin, 437
Lipohypertrophy, insulin, 338f
Lipoid proteinosis, 374f–375f
Lipoma, 429f
  multiple, 429f
Livedo racemosa, 562f
Livedo reticularis, 562f
Livedoid vasculopathy, 563f
Lobomycosis, 225f
Lobules, of subcutaneous fat, 5f
Loiasis, 298f
Loose anagen hair syndrome, 519f
Lower face acne, in adult woman, 174f
LP. see Lichen planus (LP).
Lucio phenomenon, 239, 250f
LUMBAR syndrome, 415f
Lung cancer
  hypertrophic osteoarthropathy from, 434f
  metastases, 432f–433f
Lupus erythematosus
  discoid, 23f, 101f–103f
    generalized, 103f
  hypertrophic, 17f, 103f

  neonatal, 105f–106f
    with scarring, 106f
  oral, 108f–109f
  postinflammatory hyperpigmentation secondary to, 584f
  subacute, in complement deficiency disorder, 62f
  systemic, 25f
  tumid, 104f–105f
Lupus patient, disseminated *Mycobacterium marinum* infection in, 235f
Lupus pernio, 488f–489f
Lupus profundus, 104f
  with resultant atrophy, 104f
Lupus vulgaris, 230f–232f
Lymphangiectasia, acquired, 410f
Lymphangitis, sclerosing, 37f
Lymphedema, obesity-related, 581f
Lymphocytic Sweet syndrome, 94f
Lymphogranuloma venereum, 202f
Lymphoid hyperplasia, cutaneous, 501–516
  bandlike T-cell pattern, 502f
  nodular B-cell pattern, 501f
Lymphoma
  B-cell lymphoma. see B-cell lymphoma.
  gamma delta, 512f
  secondary cutaneous, 513f
  T-cell lymphoma. see T-cell lymphoma.
Lymphomatoid papulosis, 509f–510f

M

Macroglossia, in amyloidosis, 362f
Macrophage/monocyte disorders, 479–499
Maculae ceruleae, 301f
Macular amyloidosis, 363f
Macule, labial melanotic, 464f
Maffucci syndrome, 409f
Majocchi granuloma, 206f
Major aphthous stomatitis, 558f
Mal de Meleda, 149f
Malignant lymphomas, 501–516
Mammary duct, 3f
Mammary glands, secretory portion of, 3f
Marasmus, 328f
Marfan syndrome, 351, 357f
Marginal mandibular nerve, 13f
Marginal plaque, collagenous and elastic, of hands, 148f
Mast cell, 8f
Mastocytoma
  Darier sign, 425f–426f
  solitary, 425f
Mastocytosis, 426f
  generalized adult, 427f
Median nail dystrophy, 535f
Median rhomboid glossitis, 549f
Mee lines, 533f
Melanoacanthoma, 467f
Melanocytosis, dermal, 475f–476f
Melanoma, 471f, 541f, 553f
  acral, 473f
  amelanotic, 474f
    metastatic, 475f
  color variegation, 26f
  large, 474f
  lentigo maligna, 472f
  metastatic, 475f
  nodular, 474f
  oral, 473f

Melanoma (Continued)
    satellite metastases from, 475f
    superficial spreading, 472f
    tumor, 18f
Melanonychia, longitudinal, secondary to junctional nevus, 467f
Melanonychia striata
    benign, 537f
    caused by melanoma in situ, 537f
Melanosis
    diffuse, in metastatic melanoma, 475f
    penile, 465f
    vulvar, 464f
Melasma, 584f
Melkersson-Rosenthal syndrome, 547f
Melolabial crease, 10f
Meningococcemia, 198f
Menkes kinky hair syndrome, 524f
Mental foramen, and related structures, 13f
Mercury granuloma, from thermometer, 38f
Mercury toxicity, 84f
Merkel cell, 8f
Merkel cell carcinoma, 449f
Mesenchyme, in early spine formation, 1f
Metabolism, errors in, 361–378
Metastases
    lung cancer, 432f–433f
    male breast cancer, 432f
    prostate cancer, 433f
    uterine cancer, 433f
Metastatic breast cancer, alopecia neoplastica from, 523f
Metastatic tuberculosis, 233f
Methotrexate-induced oral ulcers, 82f
Methotrexate-induced vascular hyperpigmentation, 81f
Michelin tire baby, 430f
Microcystic lymphatic malformation, 409f
Miescher granuloma, 485f
Milia, 461f
Milia en plaque, 461f
Miliaria crystallina, 28f
Miliaria pustulosa, secondary to childbirth, 29f
Miliaria rubra, 28f–29f
Milker nodule, 274f
Minocycline hyperpigmentation, 79f–80f, 554f
Minocycline pigmentation, 176f
Minocycline-induced photosensitivity, 77f
Mixed connective tissue disease, 116f
    Raynaud phenomenon secondary to, 561f
Modiolus, elevators, and depressors, 12f
Mold infections, 203
Moll glands, in eyelid, 4f
Molluscoid pseudotumor, 356f
Molluscum contagiosum, 275f–276f
Molluscum dermatitis, 276f
Mondor disease, 567f
Monilethrix, 525f
Mononucleosis, 271f
Morgellans disease, 21f
Morphea, 112f
    generalized, 112f
    with lichen sclerosis overlap, 112f
    linear, 113f–114f
Mucinoses, 119–124
    benign follicular, 122f–123f
    focal cutaneous, 124f
    follicular, associated with mycosis fungoides, 123f
    reticular erythematous, 122f
Mucinous papules, 121f
Mucocele, 556f
Mucocutaneous leishmaniasis, 293f
Mucormycosis, 225f
Mucous membranes, diseases of, 543–559
Muehrcke lines, 533f
Muir Torre syndrome, sebaceous adenomas of, 450f
Mulberry molar, congenital syphilis with, 259f
Multicentric reticulohistiocytosis, 495f–496f
Multiple carboxylase deficiency, 326f
Multiple endocrine neoplasia type 1 angiofibromas, 347f
Multiple mucosal neuroma syndrome, 428f
Mycetoma, 224f–225f
Mycobacterial diseases, 229–237
Mycobacterium abscessus infection, 236f
Mycobacterium avium-intracellulare infection
    cutaneous, 237f
    generalized, 237f
Mycobacterium chelonae infection, 236f–237f
Mycobacterium fortuitum infection, 235f–236f
Mycobacterium haemophilum cellulitis, 235f
Mycobacterium kansasii infection, cutaneous, 237f
Mycobacterium marinum infection, 233f–234f
    disseminated, in lupus patient, 235f
    in sporotrichoid pattern, 234f–235f
Mycoplasma infection, Stevens-Johnson syndrome secondary to, 74f
Mycosis fungoides, 24f
    alopecia mucinosa associated with, 507f
    follicular, 507f
    palmar plantar, 506f
    patch stage, 502f–504f
        with poikiloderma, 504f
    plaque stage, 504f–505f
    tumor stage, 505f–506f
Myelogenous leukemia cutis, acute, 515f
Myelomonocytic leukemia, 515f
    cutis, acute, 514f
Myiasis, 301f
Myrmecia, 285f
Myxedema, 119, 343f–344f
    preradial, 346f
    pretibial, 344f–345f
Myxoid cyst, 124f

N

Nail, Darier disease of, 531f
Nail dystrophy
    median, 535f
    nail patella syndrome with, 534f
    with washboard nail, 535f
Nail groove, from mucous cyst, 26f
Nail lichen planus, 529f–530f
Nail patella syndrome, 534f
    with nail dystrophy, 534f
Nail pemphigus vulgaris, 311f
Nail pits, in psoriatic nail, 530f
Nail polish, eyelid dermatitis secondary to, 71f
Nail psoriasis, 131f
    in patient with psoriatic arthritis, 530f
Nail units, examination of, 517
Nasal ala, 10f
Nasal glioma, 428f
Nasal tip, 10f
Nasoalar crease, 10f
Nasofacial sulcus, 10f
Natural killer T-cell lymphoma, 512f
Neck, posterior triangle of, anatomy of, 13f
Necrobiosis lipoidica, 375f–376f
Necrobiotic xanthogranuloma, 485f–486f
    with upper and lower eyelid involvement, 486f
Necrolysis, toxic epidermal, 21f
Necrolytic acral erythema, 272f–273f
Necrosis
    intravenous extravasation with, 79f
    subcutaneous fat, of newborn, 334f–335f
Necrotizing livedo, 563f
Neonatal cephalic pustulosis, 169, 169f
Neonatal lupus erythematosus, 105f–106f
    with scarring, 106f
Neoplasms
    epidermal, 437–462
    melanocytic, 463–477
Nephrogenic systemic fibrosis, 116f
Nerve enlargement, in leprosy, 241f
Netherton syndrome, 391f–392f
    trichorrhexis invaginata in, 525f
Neurilemmoma, 428f
Neurocutaneous diseases, 41–51
Neurofibroma, solitary, 427f
Neurofibromatosis, 18f, 383f
    with axillary freckling, 15f, 384f
    with café-au-lait macule, 384f
    with malignant peripheral nerve sheath tumor, 385f
    with plexiform neurofibroma, 384f
    segmental, 385f
Neuroma, 428f
Neuropathic ulcer
    of the hand, 51f
    in leprosy, 247f
Neutrophilic dermatosis, of dorsal hand, 94f
Neutrophilic eccrine hidradenitis, 82f
Nevi/nevus, 468f
    acral, junctional, 467f
    anemicus, 406f
    Becker, 466f–467f
    blue, 477f
    on breast, 469f
    congenital, 469f–470f
    dysplastic, 471f
    epidermal, 437–462, 437f–438f
    in genital area, 468f
    halo, 469f
    intradermal, 467f–468f
    junctional, 467f
    lipomatosis superficialis, 429f
    melanocytic, 463–477
    ocular, 468f
    oral blue, 468f
    simplex, 406f–407f
    spindle cell, 471f
    spitz, 470f
Nevus comedonicus, 438f
Nevus depigmentosus, 16f
Nevus of Ota, 15f, 476f
Nevus sebaceous, 449f–450f
    syringocystadenoma papilliferum in, 455f
Nevus spilus, 463f
New World leishmaniasis, 291f–293f
Nickel dermatitis, 69f

Nicotine stomatitis, 547f
Nipple eczema, in atopic child, 58f
Nipple skin, 3f
Nocardia, 195f
Nodular amyloidosis, 364f–365f
Nodular sarcoidosis, 487f
Nodular scabies, 304f
Nodules, weathering, 32f
Noma, 557f
Nonbullous congenital ichthyosiform erythroderma, 390f
Noninfectious immunodeficiency disorders, 53–64
Nonkeratinizing epithelium, 5f
Noonan syndrome, 381f
Normal digit, 115f
North American blastomycosis, 220f–221f
Nose
    fibrous papule of, 422f
    lateral ridge of, 10f
Notalgia paresthetica, 50f
Nummular eczema, 59f
Nutritional diseases, 323–330
    acrodermatitis enteropathica as, 326f–327f
    anemia as, 328f
    carotenemia as, 330f
    iron deficiency as, 328f
    kwashiorkor as, 328f–330f
    marasmus as, 328f
    multiple carboxylase deficiency as, 326f
    pellagra as, 325f–326f
    phrynoderma as, 323f
    scurvy as, 324f–325f
    vitamin B deficiencies as
        atrophic tongue in, 323f
        perléche in, 324f

O

Oat cell carcinoma-associated pigmentation, 555f
Obesity-related lymphedema, 581f
Occipital artery, 13f
Occipital vein, 13f
Oil burn, hot, 28f
Old World leishmaniasis, 291f
Older skin, skin tension lines in, 8f
Olmsted syndrome, 148f
Onchocerciasis, 298f–299f
Onchocercoma, 299f
Onychogryphosis, 532f
Onycholysis, 535f
Onychomadesis
    after hand-foot-mouth disease, 533f
    after toxic epidermal necrolysis, 533f
Onychomatricoma, 540f
Onychomycosis, 209f
Onychopapilloma, 540f
Onychophagia, 534f
Onychoschizia, 534f
Open comedones, 170f–171f
Oral candidiasis, 210f
Oral Crohn disease, 546f
Oral erythema, reactive arthritis with, 134f
Oral florid papillomatosis, 551f
Oral hairy leukoplakia, 17f, 551f
Oral lichen planus, 158f
Oral lichenoid dermatitis, 70f
Oral lupus erythematosus, 108f–109f
Oral lymphatic malformation, 409f

Oral melanosis, 555f
Oral melanotic macule, 554f
Oral nevus, 553f
Oral pemphigus vulgaris, 310f
Oral wart, 284f
Orf, 274f
Osler-Weber-Rendu disease, 579f–580f
Osseous sarcoidosis, 490f
Osteogenesis imperfecta, 359f
Osteoma cutis, 175f, 369f

P

Pachydermodactyly, 420f
Pachydermoperiostosis, secondary to cancer, 435f
Pachyonychia congenita, 26f, 396f
Pacinian corpuscle, in volar skin, 5f
Paederus dermatitis, 302f
Paget disease
    of breast, 448f–449f
    extramammary, 449f
Pain, 15
Palisaded neutrophilic granulomatous dermatitis, 108f
Palm, herpetic infection of, 266f
Palmar crease, xanthomas of, in hepatic cholestasis, 42f
Palmar erythema, 87f
Palmar hyperhidrosis, 528f
Palmar pits, in basal cell nevus syndrome, 445f
Palmar plantar mycosis fungoides, 506f
Palmar striae xanthoma, in biliary cirrhosis, 373f
Palmoplantar pustulosis, 138f
Pancreatic panniculitis, 336f
Panhypopituitarism, 342f
Panniculitis
    annular atrophic, 337f
    cold, 335f–336f
    pancreatic, 336f
Papillary dermis, 5f
Papillitis, 543
Papillomas, oral, in Cowden syndrome, 457f
Papillomatosis
    confluent and reticulated, 140f
    neoplasms with, 437
Papillon-Lefevre syndrome, 149f–150f
Papular atopic dermatitis, 56f
Papular mucinosis, 119
    acral persistent, 121f
    self-healing, 121f
Papular sarcoidosis, 486f–487f
Papuloerythroderma of Ofuji, 137f
    with deck chair sign, 44f
Papulonecrotic tuberculid, 233f
Papulopustular rosacea, 180f–181f
Papulosquamous diseases, 139–151
Paracoccidiomycosis, 221f–222f
Paraneoplastic pemphigus, 20f, 314f, 434f
Paraphenylenediamine exposure, depigmentation secondary to, 592f
Parapsoriasis
    digitate, 139f
    small plaque, 139f
Parasitic infestations, 291–307
Parasitosis, delusions of, 47f
Paronychia, chronic, 213f

Parotid duct, anatomy of, 11f
Parotid gland, anatomy of, 10f
Parry-Romberg syndrome, 114f
Passion purpura, 567f
Pearly penile papules, 422f
Pediatric eosinophilic pustular folliculitis, 137f
Pediculosis, 300f
Pediculosis capitis, 300f
Pediculosis corporis, 300f
Pediculosis pubis, 301f
Pellagra, 325f–326f
Pembrolizumab-associated vitiligo, 83f
Pemphigoid, bullous
    erosion, 22f
    vesicles and bullae, 19f
Pemphigoid gestationis, 316f–317f
Pemphigus erythematosus, 313f
Pemphigus foliaceus, 309, 312f–313f
Pemphigus vegetans, 309, 311f–312f
Pemphigus vulgaris, 309, 309f–311f
Penicillamine elastopathy, 354f
Perforating collagenosis, reactive, 529f
Perforating disorder, of renal failure, 529f
Perianal fissure, 22f
Perianal streptococcal infection, 192f
Perianal tinea, 207f
Perichondrium, in skin of ear, 2f
Perioral dermatitis, 182f
Periungual warts, 282f
Perléche, 210f
    in vitamin B deficiencies, 324f
Pernio, 29f–30f
Pesticide burn, 66f
Petrolatum, extraction of larva after treating with, 301f
Peutz-Jeghers syndrome, 466f, 588f
PHACE syndrome, 415f
Phacomatosis pigmentovascularis, 405f
Phaeohyphomycosis, 224f
Phenolic depigmentation, 591f
Phenytoin-induced Stevens-Johnson syndrome, 74f
Phenytoin plus radiation-induced reaction, 75f
Philtral crest, 10f
Photo onycholysis, secondary to doxycycline, 33f
Photosensitivity, to quinine, 78f
Phrynoderma, 323f
Physiologic oral pigmentation, 553f
Phytophotodermatitis, 33f
Piebaldism, 592f–593f
Piezogenic papules, 37f
Pigmentary changes, from arsenic, 588f
Pigmentary mosaicism, 380f
Pigmentation, disturbances of, 583–593
PIK3CA-related segmental overgrowth syndrome, 405f–406f
Pili annulati, 525f
Pili multigemini, 526f
Pili torti, 524f
Pilomatricoma, 455f–456f
Pincer nail, 536f
Pink disease, 84f
Pinta, 251–261, 261f
Piroxicam hypersensitivity, 19f
Piroxicam photosensitivity, 77f
Pitted keratolysis, 194f
Pityriasis alba, 57f
Pityriasis lichenoides chronica, 511f

Pityriasis lichenoides et varioliformis acuta, 510f
Pityriasis rosea, 139–151, 141f
　herald patch, 141f
Pityriasis rubra pilaris (PRP), 139–151, 142f–144f
　childhood, 144f
　circumscribed juvenile, 145f
　with early follicular hyperkeratosis, 142f
Pityrosporum folliculitis, 218f
Plane xanthoma, 372f
　in biliary cirrhosis, 373f
Plantar fibromatosis, 420f
Plantar pustulosis, 20f
Plantar warts, 282f
Plaque psoriasis, 125f
Plaque sarcoidosis, 487f–488f
Plasma cell cheilitis, 544f
Plasmacytoma, 514f
Platelet count, low, drug eruption in leukemic patient with, 73f
Poikiloderma, patch stage, mycosis fungoides with, 504f
Poikiloderma of Civatte, 31f
Poison ivy dermatitis, 65, 67f
Poliosis, 523f, 591f
Polyarteritis nodosa, 573f–574f
Polychondritis, relapsing, 118f
Polymorphous light eruption, 33f–34f
Pomade acne, 176f
Pompholyx, 58f–59f
Pore of Winer, 458f
Porokeratosis, 393f
　disseminated superficial actinic, 393f
Porokeratotic eccrine and osteal duct nevus, 394f
Porphyria cutanea tarda, 365f–366f
　hypertrichosis in, 366f
　sclerodemoid lesions in, 366f
Porphyrins, 361
Portuguese man of war dermatitis, 295f
Positive patch test, 66f
Postcapillary venule, in papillary dermis, 5f
Posterior auricular artery, 13f
Posterior auricular vein, 13f
Postinflammatory dyspigmentation, secondary to lupus erythematosus, 584f
Postinflammatory hypopigmentation, secondary to lip licking, 544f
Post-kala-azar dermal leishmaniasis, 294f
Post-steroid injection atrophy, 337f
Prader-Willi syndrome, skin picking in, 48f
Preadolescent acne, 171f
Pregnancy, pruritic urticarial papules and plaques of, 317f
Premelanosome, 7f
Prepuce, 4f
Preradial myxedema, 346f
Preservatives, vulvar dermatitis secondary to, 71f
Pretibial myxedema, 119, 344f–345f
Primary herpes simplex infection, 263f–264f
Primary HIV infection, 286f
Primary inoculation tuberculosis, 229f
Primary syphilis, 251f–253f
　chancre on patient's left palate, 253f
　with secondary lesions on palms, 253f
　on upper lip, 253f
Primrose allergy, finger dermatitis from, 58f

Progeria, 401f
Progressive nodular histiocytosis, 495f
Progressive symmetric erythrokeratoderma, 393f
Proliferative verrucous leukoplakia, 551f
Prostate cancer, metastases, 433f
Protein C deficiency, homozygous, 566f
Protein S deficiency, 566f
Proteus syndrome, 385f
　with connective tissue nevus, 385f
　with epidermal nevus, 385f
Proximal trichorrhexis nodosa, 524f
PRP. *see* Pityriasis rubra pilaris (PRP).
Prurigo nodularis, 42f, 46f
Prurigo pigmentosa, 43f–44f
Pruritus, 41–51
　chronic, 22f
Pruritus ani, lichen simplex chronicus in, 43f
Pseudocyst, auricular, 462f
Pseudofolliculitis barbae, 526f
Pseudohypoparathyroidism, 346f–347f
Pseudomonal infection, green nail secondary to, 196f
Pseudopelade, of Brocq, 522f
Pseudo-porphyria cutanea tarda, 366f
Pseudoscars, stellate, 32f
Pseudoxanthoma elasticum (PXE), 351, 352f–353f
Pseudoxanthoma elasticum-like papillary dermal elastolysis, 354f
Psoriasis, 17f, 125–138, 127f–130f
　annular, 133f
　erythrodermic, 134f
　guttate, 132f
　in HIV-infected patient, after zoster, 133f
　infantile, 131f–132f
　inverse, 131f
　linear, 132f
　nail, 131f
　　oil spot and subungual hyperkeratosis in, 131f
　nail pitting in, 130f
　pustular, 133f
Psoriatic arthritis, 134f
　nail psoriasis in patient with, 530f
Psoriatic erythroderma, 151f
Psoriatic nail
　hyperkeratosis in, 530f
　nail pits in, 530f
　oil spot in, 530f
Psychogenic excoriations, 47f
Psychogenic purpura, 568f
Pterygium inversum unguis, 535f
Pterygium unguis, 535f
Punctate keratoderma, 146f
Purple toe, secondary to cholesterol emboli, 563f
Purpura
　after vomiting, 567f
　from coin rubbing, 567f
　cough-induced, 567f
　Henoch-Schönlein, 570f
　immune thrombocytopenic, 564f–565f
　in old age, 564f
　passion, 567f
　psychogenic, 568f
　racquetball-induced, 567f
　thrombotic thrombocytopenic, 565f
　Waldenström hypergammaglobulinemic, 565f
Purpura annularis telangiectodes, 568f

Purpura fulminans, 565f–566f
Purpuric glove-sock syndrome, 280f
Pustular dermatitis, 125–138
Pustular psoriasis, 133f
PXE. *see* Pseudoxanthoma elasticum (PXE).
Pyoderma faciale, 182f
Pyoderma gangrenosum, 22f, 95f
　early, 95f
　healing, 95f
　in HIV-infected patient, 95f
Pyogenic granuloma, 18f, 412f–413f, 556f
　with satellite lesions, 413f
Pyostomatitis vegetans, 546f

Q

Quinidine photo-induced livedo reticularis, 78f
Quinine, photosensitivity to, 78f

R

Racquet nails, 534f
Racquetball-induced purpura, 567f
Radiodermatitis, chronic, 35f
Ranula, 557f
RASA1-associated capillary malformation, due to arteriovenous malformation syndrome, 408f
Raynaud phenomenon, 561f
Reactive arthritis, 135f–136f
　with conjunctival erythema, 135f
　with oral erythema, 134f
　with urethral inflammation, 135f
Reactive perforating collagenosis, 352f
Recalcitrant palmoplantar eruptions, 125–138
Recessive dystrophic epidermolysis bullosa, 387f
Recurrent herpes simplex buttock, 266f
Recurrent herpes simplex infection, 264f–265f
Recurrent labial herpes, 266f
Recurrent palmoplantar pustulosis, 138f
Red collagen bundles, in skin of young children, 2f
Red lunula, 538f
Red pigment, in cutaneous eruption, 1
Red tattoo reaction, 38f
Reeve sign, 24f
Relapsing polychondritis, 118f
Renal failure
　acquired perforating disease in, 41f–42f
　perforating disorder of, 529f
Reticular dermis, 5f
Reticular erythematous mucinosis, 122f
Reticulate acropigmentation of Kitamura, 586f
Reticulohistiocytoma, 495f
Reticulohistiocytosis
　congenital self-healing, 496f
　multicentric, 495f–496f
Retronychia, 536f
Rheumatoid nodules, 117f
Rheumatoid vasculitis, 117f
Rhinoscleroma, 199f
Rhizopus infection, 226f
Rickettsial pox, 201f
Rocky Mountain spotted fever, 200f
Romana sign, in Chagas disease, 294f

Rosacea, 169
  edema from, 181f
    by topical steroids, 182f
Rosai-Dorfman disease, 516f
Rothmund-Thomson syndrome, 403f
Rubber dermatitis, 70f
Rubella, 278f
Rubeola (measles), 277f–278f
Russell spider bite, 307f

S

Sarcoid
  annular genital, 488f
  in tattoo, 493f
Sarcoidosis, 16f, 479, 489f, 491f
  alopecia in, 492f
  annular, 488f
  digital, 490f
  erythema nodosum-like, 491f
  erythrodermic, 492f
  genital, 488f
  hypopigmentation overlying, 490f
  ichthyosiform, 491f–492f
  nodular, 487f
  osseous, 490f
  papular, 486f–487f
  plaque, 487f–488f
  scar, 493f
  ulcerative, 490f–491f
Scabies, 303f–305f
Scalp
  discoid lupus of, 520f
  erosive pustular dermatitis of, 522f
  layers of, 14f
  skin of, 3f
Scalp pemphigus vulgaris, 310f
Scar
  burn, 28f
  posttraumatic, 23f
Scar sarcoidosis, 493f
Scarlet fever, 190f
Scarring
  after scrofuloderma, 233f
  factitial, 49f
Scarring alopecia, secondary to discoid lupus erythematosus, 521f
Schamberg disease, 568f
Schimmelpenning syndrome, with lipodermoid of conjunctiva, 438f
Schnitzler syndrome, 96f
Sclerodactyly
  in limited scleroderma, 114f
  in systemic sclerosis, 115f
Scleredema, 122f
  calcinosis of knee in patient with, 114f
  limited, 24f
  in sclerodactyly, 114f
Sclerodermoid graft-versus-host disease, 63f–64f
Scleromyxedema, 119f–121f
  early, 119f
Sclerosing lymphangitis, 37f
Sclerotic digit, 115f
Scrofuloderma, 232f–233f
  linear scarring after, 233f
Scrotal calcinosis, 368f
Scrotum, lichen simplex chronicus of, 43f
Scurvy, 324f–325f
Sea urchin injury, 296f
Sea wasp dermatitis, 295f
Seabather eruption, 295f
Seaweed dermatitis, 296f
Sebaceous glands, in facial skin, 2f
Seborrheic dermatitis, 125–138, 125f–126f
  in HIV-positive patient, 126f
  with hyperpigmentation, 126f
  with hypopigmentation, 127f
Secondary syphilis, 253f–256f
  alopecia, 258f
  in HIV-infected patient, 255f
  Kaposi sarcoma and, 255f
  mucous patch, 256f
  of tongue, 256f
Segmental neurofibromatosis, 385f
Self-healing papular mucinosis, 121f
Senna burn, 66f
Sepsis, candidal, 214f–215f
Serum sickness-like reaction, 81f
Severe acne, 172f–173f
Severe infantile acne, 170f
Severe truncal acne, 173f
  with hyperpigmentation, 173f
Sézary syndrome, 508f–509f
Silica granuloma, 39f
Silicone granuloma, 38f
Sitosterolemia, 373f
Sjogren syndrome, 117f
  annular erythema of, 117f
Sjögren-Larsson syndrome, 392f
Skin
  axillary, 3f
  breast, 3f
  ear, 2f
  ear canal, 2f
  facial, 2f
    innervation of, 12f
    major anatomic landmarks in, 10f
  nipple, 3f
  older skin, skin tension lines in, 8f
  structure and function of, 1–14
  volar, 4f–5f
  in young children, 2f
Skin appendages, disease of, 517–541
Skin biopsies, for connective tissue disease, 101
Skin disease
  cutaneous signs and diagnosis of, 15–26
  diagnosis of, based on skin structure and function, 1
Skin fragility, isotretinoin, 22f
Skin lesion
  in systemic lupus erythematosus, 109f
  viral diseases and, 263
Skin picking, in Prader-Willi syndrome, 48f
Skin tag, 3f
Skin-popping ulcer, 38f
SLE. see Systemic lupus erythematosus (SLE).
Small hairs, in skin of young children, 2f
Small plaque parapsoriasis, 139f
Smallpox scarring, 274f
Smooth muscle, in breast skin, 3f
Smooth muscle hamartoma, 431f
Snake bite, 307f
Sneddon syndrome, 562f
Soft corn, 36f
Solar damage, chronic, 32f
Solar elastosis, of the forehead, 32f
Solar lentigo, 464f
Solar urticaria, 34f, 98f
Solid facial edema, 175f
Solitary congenital myofibroma, 421f
Spider angioma, 410f
Spider bite, 307f
Spindle cell hemangioma, 417f
Spindle cell nevi, 471f
Spiny hyperkeratosis, of the palms, 146f
Splinter hemorrhage, 539f
Sporotrichoid pattern, *Mycobacterium marinum* infection in, 234f–235f
Sporotrichosis, 222f
  disseminated, 223f
  fixed cutaneous, 222f
Spotted lunula, 539f
Squamous cell carcinoma, 446f, 540f, 551f–552f
  Bowen disease with, 447f
Staphylococcal abscess, 187f
Staphylococcal emboli, 185f
Staphylococcal folliculitis, 20f, 186f
Staphylococcal scalded skin syndrome, 189f–190f
Stasis dermatitis, 580f–581f
Steatocystoma multiplex, 460f–461f
Stellate pseudoscars, 32f
Steroid acne, 177f
Steroids, contact allergy to, 72f
Stevens-Johnson syndrome, 74f, 90f
  dilantin-induced, 74f
  secondary to *Mycoplasma infection*, 74f
Still disease, 118f
Stings, 291–307
Stomatitis, 70f
Stratum corneum, in eyelid, 4f
Stratum lucidum, in volar skin, 4f
Strawberry tongue, 190f
Streptococcal intertrigo, 192f
Striae distensae, 358f–359f
Sturge-Weber syndrome, capillary malformation (port-wine stain) with, 407f
Subacute cutaneous lupus erythematosus, 105f
Subacute lupus erythematosus, in complement deficiency disorder, 62f
Subcorneal pustular dermatosis, 136f
Subcutaneous emphysema, 37f
Subcutaneous fat
  diseases of, 331–338
  necrosis, of newborn, 334f–335f
Subepidermal calcified nodule, 368f
Subungual exostosis, 423f
Subungual hematoma, 539f
Subungual wart, 282f
Sulfa, erythema multiforme secondary to, 88f
Sulfa allergy, in HIV-infected patient, 75f
Sunburn, 30f
Superficial lymphatic malformation, 409f
Superficial muscular aponeurotic system, 11f
Superficial temporal artery, 10f
  and vein, 13f
Superficial thrombophlebitis, 566f
Superior labial artery, 13f–14f
Supraorbital artery and vein, 13f
Supratrochlear artery and vein, 13f
Surgical gloves, contact urticaria to, 72f
Sweet syndrome, 92f–94f
  in acute leukemia, 93f
  with acute myelogenous leukemia, 92f–93f
  histocytoid, 94f

Sweet syndrome (Continued)
  in leukemia, 93f
  lymphocytic, 94f
  in patient with systemic lupus erythematosus, 93f
Swimmer itch, 296f
Sycosis barbae, 186f
Syphilis, 251–261
  congenital, 259f
    with Hutchinson teeth, 259f
    with mulberry molar, 259f
    with scars from rhagades, 260f
  primary, 251f–253f
    chancre on patient's left palate, 253f
    with secondary lesions on palms, 253f
    on upper lip, 253f
  secondary, 253f–256f
    alopecia, 258f
    in HIV-infected patient, 255f
    Kaposi sarcoma and, 255f
    of lip with mucous patch of tongue, 256f
    mucous patch, 256f
  tertiary, 258f
Syringocystadenoma papilliferum, 455f
Syringomas, 451f–452f
  chondroid, 454f
Systemic lupus erythematosus (SLE), 25f, 107f
  acute, 106f–107f
  alopecia in, 107f
  bullous, 107f–108f
  chilblain, 107f
  with dyspigmentation, 107f
Systemic sclerosis
  dyspigmentation in, 115f
  telangiectasias in, 115f
  ulceration in, 115f
Systemic symptoms, phenytoin-induced drug reaction with, 73f–74f

T

Tache noire, 201f
Tangier disease, 374f
Targetoid hemosiderotic hemangioma, 415f
TB. see Tuberculosis (TB).
T-cell lymphoma
  angioimmunoblastic, 516f
  CD30+ anaplastic, 511f
  cutaneous, 501–516
    hydroa vacciniforme-like natural killer, 512f–513f
    natural killer, 512f
    subcutaneous, 512f
Tea tree oil dermatitis, 67f
Telangiectasia
  generalized essential, 410f
  in systemic sclerosis, 115f
  unilateral nevoid, 411f
Temporal arteritis, 576f
Tendinous xanthomas, 371f
Teratoma, 431f
Terry nail, 534f
Tertiary syphilis, 258f
Thermal burn, from child abuse, 27f
Thrombophlebitis, superficial, 566f
Thrombotic thrombocytopenic purpura, 565f
Thrush, 203
  in chronic mucocutaneous candidiasis, 210f

Thyroglossal duct cyst, 462f
Thyroid acropachy, 346f
Tick bite, 303f
Tinea, 203
  one hand involvement with, 209f
Tinea amiantacea, 528f
Tinea barbae, 204f
Tinea capitis, 203, 203f
Tinea corporis, 25f, 203, 205f
Tinea cruris, 206f
Tinea faciei, 203, 205f
Tinea imbricata, 206f
Tinea nigra, 215f
Tinea pedis, 207f–208f
  bullous, 208f
Tinea versicolor, 215f–217f
Tongue biting, chronic, fibroma secondary to, 47f
Tonofibrils, 7f
Topical antibiotic, allergy to, 72f
Topical steroid-induced atrophy, 84f–85f
Topical steroids, allergic contact cheilitis to, 543f
Torus mandibularis, 548f
Torus palatinus, 547f
Toxic epidermal necrolysis, 75f, 90f
  to Lamictal, 74f–75f
Toxic erythema, of chemotherapy, 82f
Toxicodendron dermatitis, 65
Toxin-mediated conditions, 185
Toxoplasmosis, 294f
Trachyonychia, 532f
  with koilonychia, 531f
Traction alopecia, 522f–523f
Transient acantholytic dermatosis, 322f
Transient neonatal pustular melanosis, 587f–588f
Transverse facial artery and vein, 13f
Transverse leukonychia, 536f
Transverse nail bands, secondary to chemotherapy, 537f
Triatome bite, 294f
Trichilemmoma, 457f
Trichodysplasia spinulosa, 285f
Trichoepithelioma, 456f–457f
Trichofolliculoma, 456f
Trichomycosis axillaris, 528f
Trichorhinophalangeal syndrome, 404f
Trichorrhexis invaginata, in Netherton syndrome, 525f
Trichostasis spinulosa, 527f
Trichothiodystrophy, 402f
Trichotillosis, 50f, 519f–520f
Trichrome vitiligo, 591f
Trigeminal trophic syndrome, 51f
Tropical immersion foot, 30f
Trunk, skin tension lines in, 9f
TS. see Tuberous sclerosis (TS).
Tuberculoid leprosy, 239, 240f
  borderline, 241f–243f
  early, 239f
Tuberculosis (TB), 229
  metastatic, 233f
  primary inoculation, 229f
  verrucosa cutis, 229f–230f
Tuberoeruptive xanthomas, biliary cirrhosis and, 372f
Tuberous sclerosis (TS)
  with angiofibromas, 381f
  with ash leaf macule, 382f

  with dental enamel pit, 383f
  with fibrous forehead plaque, 382f
  with paintbrush-type white streaks, 382f
  with periungual fibromas, 382f
  with shagreen plaque, 382f
Tuberous xanthomas, 370f–371f
Tufted angioma, 416f
Tufted folliculitis, 522f
Tularemia, 200f
Tumid lupus erythematosus, 104f–105f
Tumor necrosis factor inhibitor-related psoriasiform reaction, 83f
Tumoral calcinosis cutis, 369f
Tumors
  dermal and subcutaneous, 405–435
  dermal duct, 453f
  of follicular infundibulum, 459f
  giant cell, of tendon sheath, 421f
  granular cell, 405, 427f
    multiple, 427f
Tungiasis, 303f
Turner syndrome, with congenital lymphedema, 381f
Tylosis, with lung cancer, 147f
Type A pigmentary demarcation, 583f
Type B pigmentary demarcation, 583f
Type B syndrome, 348f–349f
Type C pigmentary demarcation, 583f
Type I hyperlipidemic eruptive xanthoma, 370f

U

Ulceration
  dermatomyositis with, 112f
  in systemic sclerosis, 115f
Ulcerative herpes simplex, 268f
  in HIV-infected patient, 287f
Ulcerative sarcoidosis, 490f–491f
Ulceronecrotic Mucha-Habermann disease, 510f
Ulcers
  Buruli, 235f
  factitial, 48f–49f
  neuropathic, in leprosy, 247f
Ulerythema ophrogenes, 404f
Uncombable hair syndrome, 525f
Unilateral nevoid telangiectasia, 579f
Urethral inflammation, reactive arthritis with, 135f
Urticaria, 77f, 87–99, 96f–97f
  cholinergic, 97f–98f
  cold, 97f
  delayed pressure, 98f
  exercise-induced, 97f
  solar, 34f, 98f
Urticaria multiforme, 90f
Urticaria pigmentosa, 426f
Urticarial bullous pemphigoid, 315f–316f
Urticarial vasculitis, 571f
Uterine cancer, metastases, 433f

V

Vaccinia vaccination, 274f
Varicella, 268f–269f
Vascular tumors, 405

Vasculitis
  cryoglobulinemic, 565f, 571f
  drug-induced antineutrophil cytoplasmic antibody-positive, 574f
  leukocytoclastic, 569f
  urticarial, 571f
Vasculopathy
  cutaneous collagenous, 579f
  levamisole-induced, 575f–576f
  livedoid, 563f
Vegetating pyoderma, 188f
Vemurafenib, radiation recall induced by, 82f
Venolymphatic malformation, 410f
Venous lakes, 410f
Venous malformation, 408f
Vermillion border, 10f
Verruca vulgaris, 17f
Verruciform xanthoma, 374f
Verruga peruana, 200f
Vesicular bullous pemphigoid, 316f
Vibrio vulnificus infection, 199f
Viral diseases, 263–289
Vitamin B deficiencies
  atrophic tongue in, 323f
  perléche in, 324f
Vitamin K injection site reaction, 78f
Vitiligo, 15f, 589f–591f
  granulomas in, common variable immunodeficiency with, 61f
  with koebnerization, 591f
  poliosis in, 591f
  segmental, 589f
  trichrome, 591f

Volar skin, 4f–5f
Vomiting, purpura after, 567f
Voriconazole phototoxicity, 77f
Voriconazole-induced lentigines, 15f
Vulva, lichen simplex chronicus of, 43f
Vulvar dermatitis, 71f
Vulvovaginal-gingival syndrome, 158f

W

Waldenström hypergammaglobulinemic purpura, 565f
Warfarin-induced necrosis, 78f
Warts, 281f
  in DOCK8 immunodeficiency, 61f–62f
WAS. *see* Wiskott-Aldrich syndrome (WAS).
Washboard nails
  nail dystrophy with, 535f
  secondary to habitual trauma to the matrix, 46f
Wasp sting, 302f
Weathering nodules, 32f
Wells syndrome, 92f
Werner syndrome, 400f
White dermatographism, 56f
White sponge nevus, 552f–553f
Winter itch, 43f
Wiskott-Aldrich syndrome (WAS), eczema in, 60f
Wooly hair, 526f

X

Xanthelasma, 372f
Xanthoma disseminatum, 494f
Xanthomas
  eruptive, 16f
  in homozygous familial hypercholesterolemia, 17f
  palmar, hepatic cholestasis, 42f
Xeroderma pigmentosum, 401f–402f
Xerotic eczema, 59f
X-linked ichthyosis, 21f, 389f

Y

Yaws, 251–261, 260f
Yeasts, diseases resulting from, 203–227
Yellow nail syndrome, 539f
Yellow pigments, in cutaneous eruption, 1

Z

Zeiss glands, in eyelid, 4f
Zidovudine pigmentation, 538f
Zoon balanitis, 448f
Zosteriform lentiginous nevus, 463
Zygomycosis, 203, 226f
Zyplast granuloma, 39f